10/20/15
$41.00

P9-DTN-349

THE HARSH REALITIES
OF ALZHEIMER'S CARE

THE HARSH REALITIES OF ALZHEIMER'S CARE

An Insider's View of How People with Dementia Are Treated in Institutions

ANDREW S. ROSENZWEIG, MD, MPH

The Praeger Series on Contemporary Health and Living
Julie K. Silver, MD, Series Editor

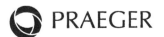 PRAEGER

AN IMPRINT OF ABC-CLIO, LLC
Santa Barbara, California • Denver, Colorado • Oxford, England

Library of Congress Cataloging-in-Publication Data

Rosenzweig, Andrew S.
  The harsh realities of Alzheimer's care : an insider's view of how people with dementia are treated in institutions / Andrew S. Rosenzweig.
      p. ; cm. — (The praeger series on contemporary health and living)
  Includes bibliographical references and index.
    ISBN 978–0–313–39890–2 (hardback : alk. paper) — ISBN 978–0–313–39891–9 (ebook)
I. Title. II. Series: Praeger series on contemporary health and living. 1932–8079
[DNLM: 1. Alzheimer Disease–psychology. 2. Attitude of Health Personnel. 3. Caregivers–psychology. 4. Long-Term Care. 5. Quality of Life. WT 155]
616.8′3–dc23   2012014834

ISBN: 978–0–313–39890–2
EISBN: 978–0–313–39891–9

16 15 14 13 12   1 2 3 4 5

This book is also available on the World Wide Web as an eBook.
Visit www.abc-clio.com for details.

Praeger
An Imprint of ABC-CLIO, LLC

ABC-CLIO, LLC
130 Cremona Drive, P.O. Box 1911
Santa Barbara, California 93116-1911

This book is printed on acid-free paper ∞

Manufactured in the United States of America

CONTENTS

Series Foreword

Contemporary Health and Living

Over the past 100 years, there have been incredible medical breakthroughs that have prevented or cured illness in billions of people and helped many more improve their health while living with chronic conditions. A few of the most important twentieth century discoveries include antibiotics, organ transplants, and vaccines. The twenty-first century has already heralded important new treatments including such things as a vaccine to prevent human papillomavirus from infecting and potentially leading to cervical cancer in women. Polio is on the verge of being eradicated worldwide, making it only the second infectious disease behind smallpox to ever be erased as a human health threat.

In this series, experts from many disciplines share with readers important and updated medical knowledge. All aspects of health are considered including subjects that are disease specific and preventive medical care. Disseminating this information will help individuals to improve their health, and that of loved ones, as well as help researchers to determine where there are gaps in our current knowledge, and help policy makers to assess the most pressing needs in healthcare.

Series Editor Julie K. Silver, MD
Assistant Professor
Harvard Medical School
Department of Physical Medicine and Rehabilitation

ACKNOWLEDGMENTS

Had I not attended the three-day Harvard Medical School course Publishing Books, Memoirs, and other Creative Non-Fiction, this book would likely never have been written. Julie Silver, MD, and her colleagues have put together a terrific annual course that I highly recommend. It was in fact at that course that my editor-to-be Debbie Carvalko heard my 90-second pitch and responded favorably to my idea and conviction. Debbie never hesitated in her enthusiasm and support, and she never once made me feel like the inexperienced first time author that I am. Her intuition and commonsense style were most appreciated, and her ideas and suggestions were spot-on.

Eugene Gallagher, Rosemary Park Professor of Religious Studies at Connecticut College, was more than generous with his time in agreeing to read and comment on an early version of the manuscript. Named Connecticut Professor of the Year in 2003 and founder of the college's Center for Teaching and Learning, Gene gave me both constructive feedback and the confidence to continue to move forward at a time when I needed someone of his stature to do just that.

My parents Fred and Marcia were, as always, incredibly supportive. They were able to find just the right balance between acknowledging how tough this was for me and encouraging me with their unique style of loving parental pressure. On a similar family note, my brothers Lance and Russ deserve more than just a passing mention. As business leaders and successful entrepreneurs, they shared their perspectives and advice on matters such as writing with an underlying mission of offering useful tips and strategies to deal with such a difficult illness. My son Jonathan was so patient and understanding of my having to miss more than a few sporting events because of this book, and for me there was no better reward for writing than the prospect of running down to the basement with him for some intense ping-pong breaks.

Speaking of dealing with this tragic disease, I'll never forget how my father-in-law Herb Weinman devoted himself selflessly to caring for his wife Elaine after she developed Alzheimer's disease several years ago. Despite the obvious toll caregiving was taking on him, he never once complained. He also never asked for help, and I hope this book benefits people who are similarly disinclined to ask for help. The experience of seeing firsthand how this illness robbed my mother-in-law Elaine of her intellect, her many talents, and her remarkable ability to give smart advice to all of her six children was always in the background during the three years of writing this book.

Finally, my wife Susan Weinman was unwavering in her positive attitude and support of my writing this book. It's not every day that the author of a book on dementia care has a wife who has not only lived through her beloved mother's Alzheimer's disease, but who is also a neurologist who is loved and respected by her patients and their caregivers. Most authors count on their spouse for patience and support, putting up with occasional weekend trips to hotels to focus on writing. I counted on her for all that and then some: exploring her observations in the long-term care facilities she visits, learning how neurologists view the world of plaques and tangles, and hearing how her patients' caregivers cope with their loved ones' dementia.

Introduction: Hidden Needs in Dementia Care Today

In part because of the terrible nature of dementia, which strips a person of his or her memories and dignity, I strongly believe I can contribute in a meaningful way to alleviating the suffering and distress that dementia causes. Consider a letter I received from the daughter of a nursing home resident with dementia that I treated recently. (I have changed their names to protect their privacy, as is true for all cases presented in this book.) Rather than emphasizing medication changes for her mother's behavior problems, I recommended that she consider moving her mother to another facility that I believed would be a better fit for her. This is something I do infrequently, in part because moving in and of itself is potentially burdensome and stressful to a person with dementia. But each nursing home has its own unique culture, its own quirks, personalities, strengths, and weaknesses. No nursing home is perfect, and it's exceedingly difficult to predict who will succeed at which particular home. But in this case, I went out on a limb and fortunately my intuition proved correct, as recounted in the following letter.

Dear Dr. Rosenzweig,

My name is Mary Smith. You had cared briefly for my mother, Mary Williams. During her evaluation at Sunny Acres Nursing Home in August 2009, you suggested she be moved as soon as possible to the Heartland Commons Nursing Home. After speaking with Dr. Clark (her attending physician) she was immediately placed on a waiting list. Six weeks later she was transferred to a much kinder facility. I had such concern about taking her to the unknown but had many sleepless nights while she was at the first location. My mom had worked many years as a nurse at a wonderful nursing home. We had never planned she would reside in one. After a seizure she was left with very little memory declaring her unsafe. As soon as she arrived to Heartland Commons she began to have some freedom, independence, and happiness return. I have such empathy for families dealing with aging parents. The use of medications and chemical restraints is more complicated than people realize. The past 20 months have been quite a journey for her. She died surrounded by a very caring staff and family.

We cannot thank you enough for helping her and so many others. I think of you often.

Our family had donations made to Heartland Commons for an educational in-service. We would like to hire you to speak to staff. Many discussions revolve around dealing with the elderly person's difficult behavior. None of us know what will become of mental health as we age. Could you speak on approaches, ideas to bring happiness, calmness, to the patients and staff? The staff was so loving and encouraged families to be involved. They are doing it right and need to know this and maybe hear some more ideas. Part of the talk could be about end of life care. There were 6 deaths in less than a week, this was very hard on the staff, many of the workers are young girls and I think this was hard for them. They do not know how valuable their loving care is.

I did follow your advice and took my mom out to my home frequently and had music at her bedside everyday. We made the best of her situation and she had a lot of fun.

Talk with the director of nursing and social worker to set a date. They will write you a check out of the fund and our family will provide some food and drinks.

Thank you so very much, it was a pleasure to meet you.

Mary Smith

Once I got over feeling flattered and proud of myself, I realized how many important messages about dementia and nursing home care were reflected in this letter, and I vowed to explore most of them in this book:

1. Alzheimer's disease has many cruel ironies: just as President Reagan, the country's Great Communicator, lost his language abilities, Mary's mother had herself worked for many years as a nurse at a nursing home.
2. Families rarely plan for their loved one to reside in a nursing home.
3. Having dementia does not mean that independence and quality of life are impossible to attain.
4. The use of medications and chemical restraints is more complicated than people realize. In April 2011, for example, the Office of Inspector General (OIG; part of the Department of Health and Human Services) released a 40-page report entitled "Medicare Atypical Antipsychotic Drug Claims for Elderly Nursing Home Residents." In it, the OIG finds that "51% of Medicare atypical antipsychotic drug claims for elderly nursing home residents were erroneous, amounting to $116 million." Yet the fact that 14 percent of 2.1 million elderly nursing home residents had at least one Medicare claim for an atypical antipsychotic drug in the first six months of 2007 shows that there is a real problem out there in managing behavior problems of people with dementia.
5. Nursing home staff are often young, inexperienced, poorly educated, and faced with very challenging work. Remarkably, despite these obstacles, many remain loving, caring, and devoted to the residents they care for.

The 36-Hour Day,[1] first published in 1981 and now in its fourth edition, is the gold standard for families and caregivers. It explains what dementia is, what symptoms accompany it, how one receives medical help for it, and what challenges affect caregivers and their loved ones. I recommend it to caregivers frequently and have read it myself. But increasingly the response I get is "Yes, I've read it " or "Yes, the Alzheimer's Association has been very helpful." But people want to go beyond the basics, beyond the traditional advice that has become commonplace. Other books address such topics as caregiver coping strategies, non-Alzheimer's dementias, person-centered dementia care, neuropsychological assessments, and scientific advances. Books have been written by patients, doctors, nurses, social workers, family members, and researchers. Aspects explored include spirituality, ethnicity, healing arts therapy, and music therapy. By reading diligently, you can apparently learn to "speak Alzheimer's," to "bathe without a battle," and to "defy dementia." You can find guidebooks that are "practical," "evidence-based," "at your fingertips," and even "for dummies." What is lacking in the field is a book that gets to the heart of understanding the hidden dementia crisis, a crisis involving numbers that are staggering: a recent report from King's College in London predicted that over 115 million people across the globe will suffer from dementia by 2050. This crisis involves the convergence of many factors: demographics, advances in medicine, social and environmental improvements, and a health care system ill equipped to handle the magnitude of the problem. In the United States, direct and indirect costs of Alzheimer's and other dementias amount to more than $148 billion annually, and, as put succinctly by the Alzheimer's Association, these illnesses "rob the nation of vast resources." Every 72 seconds, someone in America develops Alzheimer's disease; by mid-century, someone will develop Alzheimer's every 33 seconds. Why is it that a disease that affects more than 5 million people in the United States and 24 million people worldwide wreaks such havoc on individuals, systems, and institutions? Why does this disease seem to account for such a disproportionate share of distress, suffering, and chaos in our health care system? How can practical decisions be made without answers to these questions? As caregivers have become more educated and sophisticated, participating in online forums and support groups, a need exists for a more piercing look at the institutions so intimately connected with dementia care. The goal is not to blame any person, entity, institution, or funding source for the mess we are in, but to convey the "real picture" of dementia, the caregivers who live it every day. and the settings in which it is treated. Only then can we find effective ways to negotiate these various settings. Chapter 1 explores the complexity of dementia in its multiple dimensions, while Chapter 2 sheds light on my own interest and experience in the field of Alzheimer's disease. Chapter 3 delves into the concerns and importance of Alzheimer's caregivers, while Chapters 4 and 5 provide crucial insights into nursing homes and assisted living facilities, respectively. Chapter 6 addresses the importance of respite care, while Chapter 7 gives an insider's view of the inpatient psychiatric hospital. Chapter 8 focuses on memory clinics and clinical research trials, and Chapter 9 explores an issue relatively unique to dementia: mental capacity and decision making. Chapter 10 explains why workforce issues are so important to the lives of people with dementia, and Chapter 11 offers practical, sensible, and affordable strategies for caregivers and other interested parties that follow logically from the principles and examples explored. Each chapter concludes with a series of "reality lessons" based on the information presented in that chapter, lessons that are accompanied by practical strategies designed to maximize the quality of life of both the caregiver and the person with dementia.

1

THE SYNDROME OF DEMENTIA: MYTHS, MISUNDERSTANDINGS, PROGRESS, AND SETBACKS

Before we explore issues pertaining to the *settings* that people with dementia and their caregivers find themselves in, we'll pursue what may be the most serious challenge of all: the syndrome of dementia. My view is that it is the *nature of dementia itself* that largely underlies the problems we'll address in subsequent chapters.

To begin my argument, let me draw a comparison with what is arguably an equally compelling public health problem: type 2 diabetes. On one level, there are many similarities: widespread underdiagnosis and undertreatment, growing numbers of affected individuals, and the contribution of both genetic and environmental factors to the cause. However, one key difference in my view is that it is much easier to understand the underlying problems in diabetes than in dementia. For example, the fundamental problem in diabetes is a failure of the pancreas to produce insulin, or the failure of the body's insulin to function properly. Ironically, researchers are now looking at the possibility that resistance to insulin (the main cause of which is being overweight or obese) is involved as a possible cause of Alzheimer's disease.

In contrast, the underlying problems in dementia are much less well understood. Of the more than 5 million Americans affected by Alzheimer's disease in 2010, only 3 million were diagnosed. Discussing results from the Dementia Demonstration Project at the July 2010 International Conference on Alzheimer's Disease, J. Riley McCarten, MD commented that "we know dementia is common and affects over 5 million Americans age 65 and older. But in fact most people [with dementia] don't have a diagnosis. It's a looming crisis, and a big part of that crisis is due to a lack of recognition, which leads to poor quality of care and more costly care."[1]

There are many reasons for so much under-recognition of Alzheimer's disease. First of all, early signs and symptoms are so subtle that they are often missed by health care providers and family members alike. If a 51-year-old man who is a successful business owner starts having trouble making decisions, few people will think of Alzheimer's disease as a likely possibility. Rather, his problems may be attributed to depression, a vitamin deficiency, substance abuse, anxiety, or attention deficit hyperactivity disorder (ADHD).

Memory loss may not appear until many months or even years after the first signs of dementia, which may be something as seemingly unrelated as becoming increasingly socially withdrawn or anxious. Social skills are often maintained early on in the disease process so that a person may easily be able to mask his or her symptoms by engaging in what appears to be normal conversation with his or her doctor. Doctors may be too rushed, focused on other medical problems, or reimbursed too little to be vigilant about early signs of dementia in their patients, and patients and caregivers are often reluctant or even afraid to acknowledge the signs and symptoms. Finally, and you'll hear a lot more about this in this book, the social stigma associated with getting a diagnosis of Alzheimer's disease may be too much for a person to bear.

THE MYSTERY OF ALZHEIMER'S DISEASE

Part of what makes dementia so challenging as a public health problem is the inherent problem of defining and characterizing it accurately. Typically we are taught that dementia is a *syndrome* that may be caused by any (or more than one) of many *diseases*. The most common of these diseases is Alzheimer's disease (AD), followed by Lewy Body disease (a type of dementia that shares features of both Alzheimer's and Parkinson's), vascular disease, Parkinson's disease, and the frontotemporal dementias (such as Pick's disease).

The idea is that dementias (of which Alzheimer's disease is the most common) are characterized by multiple cognitive deficits, share some common presentations, but have many causes. This is not as straightforward a point as it may seem; at least monthly I come across a caregiver who insists her loved one has "Alzheimer's but not dementia." While this has been the accepted teaching since the early 1990s, the reality is much more complicated. For example, consider some recent comments made by a leader in the field of dementia, Vladimir Hachinski, MD. Dr. Hachinski, professor of neurology at the University of Ontario and editor-in-chief of *Stroke*, commented in 2008 that the concept of dementia is too "categorical, exclusive, and arbitrary."[2] In his view, the diagnostic criteria are so variable that there is often no real diagnosis until "long after AD has taken hold of the brain."[3]

Even the neuropathological hallmarks of Alzheimer's, the plaques and tangles, are "fraught with problems" since many postmortem brains have plaques and tangles but the person has *no* history of the disease. He argues that since cerebrovascular disease and Alzheimer's disease share similar risk factors (i.e., hypertension, lack of exercise, unhealthy diet, smoking, etc.), "dementia is not a good way to capture AD."[4]

Zaven Khachaturian, PhD, who at the National Institutes of Health (NIH) helped set up the first federal research effort on AD, commented that Dr. Hachinski's argument reflects the holes that exist in the Alzheimer's field and that both Alzheimer's and vascular disease risk factor reduction should be targeted together. To hear such a respected figure voice the opinion that the concept of dementia is obsolete makes it easier to see why members of the general public have a hard time wrapping their arms around this illness that has so greatly impacted their lives.

To make matters worse, while the field has made significant advances in the past 10 years, the future is uncertain. Given the aging population and the increasing survival rates for persons with AD, by 2050 the number of individuals with AD who are age 85 years or older is expected to more than quadruple, from 1.8 million to 8 million. The etiology and pathophysiology remain uncertain and controversial; while the two pathological hallmarks are plaques and tangles, it remains unclear how the plaques actually damage neurons. As recently as February 2009, a link with prion proteins (which cause mad cow disease and Creutzfeld-Jakob disease) was reported. Stephen Strittmatter, one of the study's authors and the Vincent Coates Professor of Neurology at Yale University School of Medicine, stated that these proteins "seem to interact with early stage plaques in the brain in a way that allows those plaques to damage brain cells."[5]

While the study doesn't suggest that prion proteins actually cause Alzheimer's, it illustrates the wide range of possible treatments that are under discussion and development. Summarized in a January 2011 editorial in the *Journal of the American Medical Directors Association*,[6] several therapies are being developed for Alzheimer's disease. I will provide a brief summary of each proposed therapy:

1. Acetylcholinesterase inhibitors (already available as donepezil [Aricept], rivastigmine [Exelon patch], and galantamine [Razadyne]). These are medications that are already FDA-approved for the treatment of Alzheimer's disease. They increase the level of a brain chemical (neurotransmitter) called acetylcholine, which plays an important role in memory and learning. While these are core medications for Alzheimer's disease, they treat symptoms rather then modify the disease. In other words, while they may delay the progression of symptoms for 6 to 12 months in people who take them, they don't directly affect the beta-amyloid protein that is the key component of the brain plaques that many scientists believe contribute to the cause of Alzheimer's disease.
2. NMDA receptor antagonists (available as memantine [Namenda]). Memantine, a medication that is also FDA-approved for Alzheimer's disease (in the moderate to severe stages), blocks a specific receptor in the brain. This receptor, the N-methyl-D-aspartate (NMDA) receptor, can lead to the death of brain cells when overstimulated by another neurotransmitter called glutamate. Memantine works by regulating the activity of glutamate, which also plays a key role in memory and learning.

3. Preventing production of beta-amyloid. Beta-amyloid is a naturally occurring protein fragment in the brain. When it accumulates in the spaces between brain cells, however, it becomes toxic, clumping together into what is called oligomers. According to the amyloid cascade hypothesis, the leading theory that explains how Alzheimer's diseased is caused, it is these oligomers that are toxic to brain cells, causing the very early cognitive problems in Alzheimer's disease. Later, these oligomers form the plaques that are characteristic of Alzheimer's disease, but it is the oligomers as opposed to the plaques that are the actual toxic agents.

4. Increasing beta-amyloid protein clearance. Under normal circumstances, the brain eliminates most beta-amyloid. In Alzheimer's disease, however, beta-amyloid is produced in the brain at a normal rate but not cleared, or removed from the brain, efficiently. One study, for example, found that the clearance of beta-amyloid was about 30 percent slower in people with Alzheimer's disease than in cognitively normal individuals. While for years scientists believed that it was the overproduction of beta-amyloid that led to its accumulation in the brain, now the emphasis has shifted to the clearance of beta-amyloid.

5. Preventing beta-amyloid protein aggregation. The idea here is that drugs that inhibit the aggregation of beta-amyloid could protect brain cells from the toxic effect of beta-amyloid discussed previously. One class of drugs called nitrophenols is being actively studied in this regard.

6. Decreasing tau aggregation. In addition to beta-amyloid, the other most frequently mentioned protein that contributes to the cause of Alzheimer's disease is tau. While amyloid plaques are made up of beta-amyloid, neurofibrillary tangles are composed of tau proteins. Tau proteins play a crucial role in the structure of brain cells, and the tangles that they form result in the death of these brain cells. In fact, Alzheimer's disease and other types of dementias that are accompanied by tau protein aggregation are often called tauopathies.

7. Reversing mitochondrial dysfunction. The mitochondrial cascade hypothesis of Alzheimer's disease is explored in detail later in this chapter.

8. Other treatments (including testosterone and nerve growth factor [NFG]). According to John Morley, MD, director of geriatric medicine at Saint Louis University and a coinvestigator of a study on testosterone, "having low testosterone may make you more vulnerable to Alzheimer's disease," and "we should pay more attention to low testosterone, particularly in people who have memory problems or other signs of cognitive impairment."[7] As far as NGF, a study is underway with a gene therapy product called CERE-110 that is designed to deliver NGF to the brain for the treatment of Alzheimer's disease. The rationale is that NGF is known to promote survival of cholinergic brain cells that degenerate in Alzheimer's disease and may therefore provide sustained functioning of these cells.[8]

The fact that so many types of treatments are being proposed points to how elusive treatments or cures have been for Alzheimer's disease. Three notable recent failures of drugs for Alzheimer's disease are tarenflurbil (Flurizan), semagecestat, and dimebolin hydrochloride (Dimebolin). In fact, presently there are about 100 medicines in the later stages of the drug development pipeline, meaning they are either in clinical trials (see also Chapter 8) or awaiting FDA review. In addition to CERE-110 mentioned previously, I'll highlight several of the more promising drugs that are currently being tested in clinical trials:

1. Bapineuzumab. This drug is an antibody to the beta-amyloid plaques discussed previously. There are 14 ongoing clinical trials in more than 10,000 patients, and the results of some of the completed studies should be available in late 2012.
2. Gammaglobulin. This is being tested to determine if intravenous immuno-globulin (IGIV) treatment slows the rate or prevents the progression of dementia symptoms in individuals with mild-to-moderate Alzheimer's disease. The theory here is that IVIG contains antibodies against beta-amyloid.
3. Solanezumab. This drug is also a beta-amyloid antibody that is being investigated as a potential treatment to slow the progression of mild-to-moderate Alzheimer's disease.

THE MITOCHONDRIAL CASCADE HYPOTHESIS

Item number 7 in the earlier list of proposed therapies, namely reversing mitochondrial dysfunction, is worth commenting on here. In fact, the "mitochondrial cascade hypothesis" of Alzheimer's disease is a theory that has been gaining followers in explaining what causes Alzheimer's disease. As the power generators of our body's cells, mitochondria are often abnormal in people with Alzheimer's disease.

According to the mitochondrial cascade hypothesis, the key brain changes that occur in Alzheimer's disease, namely the production of amyloid plaques and neurofibrillary tangles and the death of brain cells, are actually caused by the changes in mitochondrial functioning that occur as people age. Since it is well accepted that mitochondrial functioning declines with age, the proponents of this theory see a strong connection between this age-related decline and older age as the number one risk factor for developing Alzheimer's disease. They point out that most people who live long enough will eventually develop Alzheimer's disease, and that many elderly people with plaques and tangles in their brains do not have dementia. According to their theory, a person's genes determine how durable their mitochondria are, and the rate of decline in their mitochondria determines the age at which dementia begins. Another factor that supports their hypothesis is that defects in three mitochondrial enzymes have been found in people with Alzheimer's disease. If this theory has merit, efforts at developing Alzheimer's treatments should target declining mitochondrial function, perhaps by enhancing the expression of mitochondrial genes or by finding ways to increase the aerobic metabolism of brain cells.[9]

CAN'T WE JUST COUNT THE PLAQUES AND TANGLES?

Consider an October 2009 article by Majid Fotuhi, MD, PhD. In "How Accurate Is Alzheimer's Diagnosis Among Patients Over 80?" Dr. Fotuhi argues that instead of Alzheimer's disease, multiple pathologies contribute to dementia in most people over the age of 80. He reviews the history of what memory loss in the elderly has been attributed to over time, starting with Pythagoras in the seventh century BCE, who considered it a "return to imbecility of infancy." Later theories attributed it to "normal aging," demonic possession, syphilis, strokes, hardening of the arteries, and (since the late twentieth century) to Alzheimer's disease.[10]

He cites a 2009 study in which detailed evaluations were performed on 456 elderly people who had donated their brains for the longitudinal Cognitive Function in Ageing Study. Many of the findings are "exactly opposite of what would have been expected based on the current views of late-life dementia." Amazingly, in elderly patients with dementia, the amount of plaques and tangles actually appears to *decrease* or remain constant in the hippocampus and neocortical areas (the brain regions most affected in AD), while in the elderly control group without dementia, the levels of Alzheimer's pathology *increase* with each decade of life. Instead of the plaques and tangles being the key problem, it is the degree of atrophy (shrinkage) in the hippocampus and cortex that is the variable most correlated with dementia.

Concluding his January 2011 editorial on future treatments of Alzheimer's disease, Dr. Morley notes that it has been assumed that amyloid-beta is just a toxic agent. But in fact "like thyroid hormone, it produces diseases if there is too little or too much. In addition, like diabetes mellitus there clearly is more than one type of Alzheimer's disease with multiple possible causes."[11]

BEYOND THE SCIENCE: EMOTIONS AND PSYCHOLOGY

The second part of my argument regarding why dementias are so devastating relates to the sheer *emotional and psychological burdens* to both patient and caregiver. Consider the following two pieces, one written by a person with Alzheimer's disease and one written by the 18-year-old granddaughter of a person with Alzheimer's disease.

The first was written recently by a patient of mine (V. C.) who lives in an assisted living facility (ALF), an 85-year-old widowed woman with moderate Alzheimer's disease who is convinced people are stealing her possessions and then "selling them across the street." A very proud and proper woman (during our interview she reminded me of her high level of intellect and Mensa membership), she wrote the following letter to her father, deceased for at least 20 years but very much alive and well to his daughter.

Dear Dad,
    I've been here now at the "Funny Farm." I have been feeling sick for the past 2 weeks from the pills Mom insisted I take from a Doctor I don't remember knowing—let alone consulting.
    I have had the money I came with stolen from my pocketbook, plus half my clothes stolen from my room. I no longer have a car I can use—it is still in the yard

at Altria under the snow or ice if it hasn't melted. Someone has stolen the keys to it so I can't drive it anyhow.

I'm not trying to start a fight but I agreed when you asked me to come here. However I could use a little help. I could have worked and made some money during the time I've been here. I now have an empty wallet, plus no car and a very slim wardrobe.

I'm not asking for money. I want to get out of here and I need a ride home from either you or Mom. If I could get home maybe I could find a job and make some money. I'm of no use here. This place where I'm staying at your request is going down hill in a hurry. Most of the inmates here are thieves—they steal anything they see. The food gets worse with every passing day.

Jennifer and Danielle are the only family members I've seen since I've been here and they have been long gone to go on with their lives. I have done more than any family members would.

I need a ride out of here back to my house. I need to contact a "good" Doctor to find out why I feel so tired and sick and I need to find a job so I can support myself.

I responded when you asked me to come here and now I need a little help!!!

Please call me or come to see me so we can talk. Tell Mom I want to talk to her too.

P.S. This is the second time I've written to you. I've never had a response. I guess I'm no longer a member of the family.

Just remember one thing. I'm still young; your not. You may need me sometime in the future.

I must admit I was deeply moved by this letter. The nurse at the ALF who shared it with me (in the secure dementia unit) fought back tears as we discussed it. Yet once I got past the emotional impact, I realized that in a single two-page letter, this woman illustrated as many important messages and themes about Alzheimer's disease as virtually any textbook could.

Let's examine each of the major themes that registered with me, although I'm sure there are others that I will have missed.

1. Delusions
2. Losses
3. Home
4. Driving
5. Insight
6. Resilience
7. Anger

1. Delusions

Delusional thought content is common in dementia, with most studies suggesting an incidence of 34 to 50 percent. Delusions often explain agitation and aggression, although it is often difficult to differentiate between true delusions (fixed, false beliefs) and confusion. Misplacing personal belongings, for example, can lead someone to the conclusion that his or her belongings have been stolen, and of course, sometimes their belongings *really have* been stolen. V. C.'s letter indicates that she, too, is affected by the most common delusional belief in Alzheimer's disease, the belief that people are stealing her things. That this belief is a true delusion is further emphasized by her extension of this belief into the belief that the thief is later selling her things for personal gain. While most people now know that it only makes things worse to confront the person or to argue about the truthfulness of the complaint, there are only so many times that a sane adult can answer "I'll help you find them" when his wife or mother maintains that her clothes have been stolen.

Other frequent delusions a patient with dementia has include the belief that staff and other residents are trying to hurt him or her, that his or her spouse is having an affair, and that his or her house is not his or her home. As if caring for your spouse with dementia isn't stressful enough, imagine the additional strain posed by your spouse's adamant belief that you're being unfaithful. One of my nursing home patients with a loving, devoted wife was extremely angry with her for what he described as her "sleeping with three different men down the hall." Knowing he would become enraged by her visits, she began to visit less and less frequently. Despite three psychiatric hospitalizations, numerous medication trials, and attempts at psychotherapy, his delusion persisted. The details would never be the same, yet the overall theme of unfaithfulness persisted. Two years later, only after his dementia worsened noticeably, did the delusions finally decrease in prominence, though they never disappeared completely.

Less commonly, people are convinced people on the television are real, that strangers are living with them, or that people close to them are actually impersonators. Misidentifying people is also more common than many realize. I'll never forget an ALF resident (in an Alzheimer's unit) I saw a number of years ago with a "mirror sign" delusion, that is, the inability to recognize her own reflected image. She would literally stand in front of the full-length mirror outside her room and converse with the image she saw as if it were a "friend," sharing her thoughts and making friendly conversation. After a while, the staff and the other residents just adapted to this behavior. There seemed no need to attempt to treat it with medication since it was harmless and actually seemed to enhance her quality of life by increasing her self-esteem. On the other hand, you can imagine a mirror delusion that is not so benign. If a person with Alzheimer's disease believes she is still 30 years old and expects to see that person in the mirror, the image may be extremely disconcerting and frightening. In that situation, it would make sense to remove the mirror.

Of course in chronic psychiatric illnesses like schizophrenia, delusions are part and parcel of the illness. In general, they are more bizarre and complex than the delusions in dementia. An example is the belief that the CIA or some secret government agency has been able to implant wires or a radio device into the patient's brain, which enables the agency to monitor his or her thoughts and even dictate his or her behavior and actions. But family members of schizophrenic patients have usually had many years to come to terms with their loved one's illness, to know the stigma of a mental illness, and to face a system that presents tremendous barriers to overcome. In dementia, the patient typically has no premorbid psychiatric illness, with the likely exception of depression or anxiety. Yet now, as a result of his or her dementia, he or she is *behaving like a psychiatric patient*, with delusions and possibly hallucinations that people fear and often perceive as "crazy."

The first U.S. population study of behavioral disturbances in dementia was the Cache County Study of Memory in Aging, the results of which were published in 2000.[12] The study evaluated both how common and how severe mental and behavioral disturbances in the elderly were. The study enrolled 90 percent (5,092 individuals) of the people in Cache County, Utah, that were at least 65 years of age, including about 800 people that were at least 85 years of age. The 329 individuals with dementia were compared with a group of 673 individuals without dementia, and the results were telling.

In the individuals with dementia, delusions were 8 times more frequent than in those without dementia, and hallucinations were 23 times more frequent. Similarly, agitation and aggression were 8.5 times more common in the demented individuals, while depression was more than 3 times as common. As a result of the symptoms, people with dementia often are burdened with stigma and the unfair judgments of others.

In a March 2009 study conducted by Harris Interactive, 57 percent of caregivers (out of 539 caregivers) said that the diagnosis of their loved one's Alzheimer's disease was delayed because either they were, or the person with the illness was, in denial about having the disease or feared the social stigma associated with it. Eleven percent said the patient's own shame related to the disease held the caregivers back from seeking help, while 5 percent of the caregivers said they themselves were the ones who feared the stigma. This latter group reported an average time of *6 years* between the onset of symptoms and diagnosis.[13]

2. Losses

The sheer number and types of losses in dementia are overwhelming. The third edition of the book *Understanding Dementia* devotes an entire chapter to the losses in dementia. From a cognitive sciences perspective, these losses include attention, concentration, perception, orientation, insight, judgment, memory, speech and language, mobility, and coordination.[14] But the losses that are painfully apparent to V. C. and expressed in her letter are less technical and more human: the loss of independence, of self-esteem, and of a sense of contributing to society in a meaningful way; the loss of control, of freedom, and of health. That she feels so "tired and sick" says nothing about her true physical condition: on paper she is quite healthy and takes few medications. But her life is crumbling as her brain is atrophying. Quoting from *Understanding Dementia*,

"As widespread areas of the brain are progressively damaged in dementia, the functions of these areas decline."[15] The loss of brain cells in dementia corresponds to the emotional and human losses expressed so movingly by V. C.

3. Home

Voicing a desire to "go home" is one of the most common real-life manifestations of dementia. Many Alzheimer's caregiver–oriented websites address this problem, with one of the best explanations I've discovered as follows:

> A common phrase heard from people with dementia in residential care is "I want to go home." This can be especially upsetting for families and caregivers. Wanting to go home may be caused by feelings of insecurity, depression, or fear. It may be that "home" is a term used to describe memories of a time or place that was comfortable and secure. "Home" may be memories of childhood or of a home or friends who no longer exist.[16]

Another fascinating aspect of "home" in dementia is the degree to which dementia sufferers differ in their reactions to this concept. In "Understanding the Dementia Experience,"[17] Jennifer Ghent-Fuller writes:

> Some families have described their loved ones with Alzheimer disease as engaged on a restless search for reality and "the known," which they can never find. These people are rarely happy. Many spousal caregivers describe the person with Alzheimer disease as only happy at times they are out—for a drive, to a restaurant, at the market, and so on. It may be that they are happy only when they are away from their residence, and away from the environment in which they have a sense of frustration, despair and injustice at no longer being able to function at home. There are no demands on their disappearing skills when they're out for a drive. In contrast, others with dementia have said they are only really happy and secure when they are at home and feel quite nervous when they are out. One lady would agree to go to a musical play in another city only if her name and address and that of her daughter were pinned on her coat; she knew she wouldn't be able to get herself home if they became separated in the crowd. Each individual has unique needs.

In any support group I've ever led or been a part of, I've always been asked how to deal with this request to "go home," as it so often frustrates families and professionals alike. If I had a medication I could prescribe that would make this phrase go away, I'd probably be considered a genius. But consider that instead of viewing home as "a person's usual residence," perhaps home should be viewed somewhat differently. The following is the fourth of 11 definitions of the word "home" found in the American Heritage Dictionary of the English Language: "an environment or haven of shelter, of happiness and love." I believe it is this notion that is being expressed by so many people affected by dementia, the importance of domestic affections, the value of shared and loving intimacy experienced in family life. Wanting her father to get her "a ride back to my house" is V. C.'s way of wanting to reconnect with the one part of her life that provided the most security, intimacy, and comfort.

4. Driving

Being told you are unfit to drive is often "the straw that breaks the camel's back." I've treated many patients with dementia whose emotional health held up remarkably well until the loss of driving privileges led to an episode of depression and a decline in other functional areas. While often taken for granted as a routine part of adult life, driving is a strong symbol of independence and competence. Measures taken to counter a person's unwillingness to give up driving may be extreme: replacing keys with other keys that don't work, removing the battery cable, having a "kill switch" installed.

It's when "lying, cheating, and stealing" become real options for families who are terrified of the prospect of their loved ones driving unsafely, with potentially devastating consequences. In my experience, the commonly advised notion of getting the doctor to write a prescription that says no more driving is laughable. I've never once heard of this strategy actually succeeding, and furthermore, how is it that a physician is magically able to be the arbiter of a person's driving ability? Driving behaviors really need to be observed over a reasonable period of time before one can come to a reasonable conclusion. The cognitive abilities that particularly impact driving ability include judgment, orientation, multi-tasking, reaction times, and visuospatial skills.

I've had patients with dementia who I would have bet money would be found unfit to drive, yet because of their lifelong vocations as professional drivers passed road tests with flying colors. The dementia screening test performed by most physicians, the Mini-Mental Status Examination (MMSE), was never designed to be, nor has it been validated as, a predictor of driving safety. In fact, studies have shown it to be inconclusive as a predictor of crash risk. While other tests, including the Clinical Dementia Rating Scale (CDR), the Useful Field of View test (UFOV), and the Gross Impairment Screening tool (GRIMPS), have been used for driver evaluation in dementia, it is known that cognitive tests alone are not sufficient to determine fitness to drive. An on-road driving assessment by an experienced driving evaluator is still considered the gold standard to evaluate driving abilities in people with dementia.

A significant problem is the inability to know definitively when driving should stop. While eventually everyone with Alzheimer's disease will lose the ability to drive safely, driving in mild, early stage dementia is usually not a major issue. Warning signs that a person with dementia should stop driving include failing to observe traffic signals, hitting curbs, signaling incorrectly, driving at inappropriate speeds, moving into the wrong lane, confusing the brake and gas pedals, and stopping in traffic for no apparent reason.

An excellent resource from the National Highway Traffic Safety Association that delves into these issues in more detail is available online.[18]

5. Insight

Although most people with Alzheimer's disease are unaware of their deficits, I have always been amazed at the occasional person who, despite being in the moderate stage of the disease, will matter-of-factly point out that she has Alzheimer's disease "just like my mother did." A practical definition considers insight as the ability to judge both the presence and the severity of illness. One author defined it as "the capacity to discern the true nature of the situation, or as applied to dementia, the recognition of the fact, degree, and implications of one's own illness."[19]

Individuals with dementia are often aware of some deficits but not others, and while they may be aware of a particular deficit, they may be unaware of the consequences of that deficit. I've worked with many patients who knew they had a memory problem but had no idea that they were paranoid or aggressive. Others would admit their memory was poor but would attribute it to normal aging, even when the memory loss was so severe the person couldn't remember any of three words in 15 seconds or so.

Of course, those who retain insight are probably more likely to develop depression and grief as they come to terms with the enormity of the diagnosis, although it is interesting that several studies have found that depression in Alzheimer's disease is unrelated to patient self-awareness of illness.

Another interesting aspect of the existing research on insight in dementia is that there appears to be a disproportional degree of loss of insight associated with Alzheimer's disease when compared with vascular dementia. While it makes sense to say that usually as the severity of dementia increases the awareness of the deficits decreases, the relationship is far from linear. My own experience is that for people in the mild or moderate stage of disease, it's virtually impossible to predict which patients will have awareness of their symptoms and limitations. More often than not, the phrase "she overestimates her abilities" appears in the medical chart, often as a prelude to arguing that the person is "unable to return home without 24-hour supervision." These phrases are unfortunate and illustrate some of the many systemic biases that creep into our health care system's approach to people with dementia. How is it that an emergency department physician or physical therapist who has performed an evaluation is able to state with any degree of confidence who is able to safely return home and who isn't? Unless the home situation is looked at carefully, with input from family, neighbors, and others, these decisions may amount to little more than guesswork.

While it's true that some people with Alzheimer's disease can tell when living alone is no longer safe or desirable, typically people want to stay in their own homes for as long as possible, even if there are some safety issues. In addition to lacking insight about their deficits, they may be concerned that a move away from home would mean a loss of self-reliance and control over their daily lives.

As with many aspects of dementia care, barriers within the health care, community care, and legal systems often conspire to make it challenging for family members and health care professionals to determine if a move from home is needed or if additional support can be provided in the home. These barriers include the difficulty of sharing information under privacy and confidentiality regulations, the limited availability of services to support independent living, and the complexities of the laws that determine when a person is no longer able to make certain decisions for themselves (Chapter 9 explores decision-making capacity in much more detail).

We would all likely agree that people with Alzheimer's disease need to live in environments that best support their safety and quality of life. For some, this may mean living at home with support services, even if there is some risk. No one can live a life free of risk, and if risks have been identified, it is important that family members and health care professionals try to lessen them wherever possible. For example, a person who frequently leaves the stove on should probably have his stove disconnected. There are plenty of other ways to provide hot food, such as Meals on Wheels.

Other factors to be taken into account when it comes to a person with dementia safely living alone include the following:

- Is the person able to take medication properly?
- If sick, would the person be able to understand and take appropriate action, such as calling for help?
- Is the person able to take care of personal hygiene, such as bathing and toileting?
- Are there current or past health problems that might put the person at risk of harm?
- Is the person able to eat nutritiously throughout the day?
- Is the person able to store foods properly?
- Does the person pose a risk to others? For example, does the person live in an apartment and regularly cause fires with the stove or cigarettes?
- Is the person able to react and take action in an emergency, such as a fire?
- Is the person's home safe?

Returning to the insight issue, I recall a woman I recently saw at a nursing home who would yell out intermittently but loudly whenever she was alone in her room. When I walked into her room, feeling confident that as the dementia expert I would "get to the bottom of this" and uncover the woman's unmet needs, I was told quite matter-of-factly that "I yell because I want attention."

In the case of V. C., as is true for most patients with dementia, there *is* an awareness that something is wrong. She writes in her letter that she feels "tired and sick" but would never acknowledge that she is memory impaired and paranoid.

When a person with dementia lacks insight into having a problem, it makes it much more likely that he or she will refuse medications. This creates a difficult situation in which caregivers are often tempted to conceal medications in the food or drink of a person with Alzheimer's disease. A large nursing home study in Norway found that while 95 percent of the residents had medications that were routinely put in their food or drink, only 40 percent of the patients' records made note of the surreptitious administration. As noted in a recent paper on the subject:

> Covert medication may seem like a minor matter, but it touches on legal and ethical issues of a patient's competence, autonomy, and insight. Medicating patients without their knowledge is not justifiable solely as a shortcut for institutions or families wishing to calm a troublesome patient and thus alleviate some of the burdens of care giving. The paramount principle is ensuring the well-being of a patient who lacks the competence to give informed consent. Ethically, covert/surreptitious administration can be seen as a breach of trust by the doctor or by family members who administer the drugs. Covert medication contravenes contemporary ethical practice.[20]

My experience has been that opinions differ greatly on this: many family members believe that if giving medication covertly alleviates distress, helps delay nursing home placement, or helps with medical problems like thyroid disease or high blood pressure, it is worth it. A study in England in 2000 found that of 50 people caring for people with dementia, 48 thought the practice of hiding medications in food was sometimes justified.[21] But certainly not all people feel that way.

6. Resilience

Clinical psychologist Susan McCurry offers caregivers a set of practical and flexible tools to enable them to become more resilient in the face of difficulty and change. As she writes:

> These caregivers fit a pattern that I call Resilient Caregivers. These resilient caregivers come from every age, gender, socioeconomic level, and ethnic background; they can be spouses, adult children, distant relatives, good friends, or paid staff. Despite their apparent diversity, resilient caregivers share some important commonalities. Although they are often caring for someone with significant psychiatric or physical impairment, they are able to detach themselves and not take the person's behavior personally. They maintain their sense of humor.[22]

While I agree with the notion that resilience in caregiving is extremely important in dementia, I find it curious that most of the literature on resilience in dementia refers to *caregivers* as opposed to *patients.* Now consider the first paragraph from an editorial by Phyllis Braudy Harris and John Keady:

> The concepts of wisdom, resilience and successful aging are not often spoken in the same sentence as the word dementia. In fact, many people might even think this sequencing is an oxymoron. Yet, as researchers, health/social care professionals and voluntary service personnel work more closely with people with dementia as co-researchers/inquirers and mentors, the connection of these three words to the lived experience of dementia gains increasing relevance and meaning.[23]

By definition, resilience is the ability to recover quickly from illness, change, or misfortune. So isn't it natural that the person living with the disease might possess resilience as well? In fact, I can't agree more that people with dementia are resilient. In referring to her assisted living facility as the "funny farm," in pleading with her father to let her "get home to find a job and make some money," V. C. is also showing resilience in the face of a terrible disease; even in the face of a damaged brain, her way of coping appears to be quite appropriate.

7. Anger

Anger is another near-universal feature of Alzheimer's disease and other dementias. As with V. C., it is extremely common for people with Alzheimer's disease to be looking for their parents. As the disease progresses, the person inevitably passes through his or her own childhood. Professionals and caregivers alike learn quickly that attempting to tell a person with dementia that his or her parents are long dead is both useless and deleterious, leading to distress and anger. Since the events of their parents' death are no longer part of the memory of the person with Alzheimer's, the anger stems in part from their "knowing perfectly well" that their parents are not dead.

Disinhibition is another factor that underlies anger outbursts in dementia: the controls that a person has spent a lifetime building over certain aspects of their personality are gradually eroded, and anger may erupt impulsively and explosively.

One relatively straightforward way of understanding why difficult behaviors like anger outbursts occur so often in people with dementia is to think of four basic losses that occur in thinking. In people without dementia, feelings lead to thoughts, which in turn lead to behaviors. But in dementia, that path is short-circuited at the level of thoughts. First, people lose their *memory* of how they've coped with situations in the past. Second, people lose their *judgment* to select among alternative actions. Third, people lose the *insight* needed to solve problems. And finally, people with dementia lose the *inhibitions* and *impulse control* needed to show restraint.

The second piece I'd like to share illustrates the profound emotional impact Alzheimer's disease has on family members. Danielle is a college freshman in Vermont. Since she was 8 months old, she has visited her grandparents in Texas every year. In addition, her grandparents made the trek to New England to visit Danielle and her family every summer until her grandfather, nicknamed PopPop, was placed in the Alfredo Gonzales Texas State Veterans Home in McAllen, Texas, in 2006. PopPop had in fact built and did much work on Danielle's Vermont home. Danielle wrote this as a short story for a class, titling it "The Man Who Knew Me."

A warm breeze blows across my freckle-filled face as I emerge from behind the airport doors. The palm trees sway to the beat of the breeze, *swooshing* through the dry, warm night air. Its midnight yet there isn't a chill in this night air. The warmth of a Texas night embraces my whole body, hugging my every curve, washing over me. Then the ice cold air of the Lincoln MKZ hits me flat in the face. Into my Nana's car I climb.

The lights blur by as we speed down the bump-filled road to her one-story home. I know that we are home when the sound the tires make goes from gliding over pavement to rolling over my grandma's cobblestone drive. The garage door lifts up just in time for us to pull into the drive way. My PopPop's boxes sit there, lonely and untouched, just waiting for the day when he returns home. So am I.

I open the faded door. A grey and black speeding blob races towards me. Mitzi. My Nana's built-in, fuzzy alarm system, that barks at the sound of a pin dropping, now that she lives alone. I wander through her tidy house, waiting. Waiting for him. Waiting to see his worn face and his silver white hair. Waiting to hear him call me *Danyeller.* Waiting for a hug, a hug so powerful it takes your breath away. But then I remember. I guess I'll just have to keep waiting.

Three towering flag poles frame the entrance to *the* building. The building where *he* is. The automatic doors part in front of me. I hesitate, afraid to continue. Afraid of what I will see, but more afraid of what I will not see and will never be able to see again. *Bright, vibrant blue eyes, full of life, joy, and knowledge that sparkle if you catch them in the right light. Shiny, silky white hair. An aged face framed by square glasses, still full of promise and love. The face of the man who once knew me. The face of my PopPop.*

I drift down the hallway to his wing, seemly taking days to do such a simple task. Like I am stuck in something dense and unforgiving. There it is. Standing tall in all its shininess. Taunting me. Egging me to come forward and knock. Provoking me to step through it and face the harsh reality. So I do.

All of a sudden, there I am. Standing in a room full of men and women who, at one time, put their lives on the line for this country that we reside in. People who sacrificed everything to make this country a better place for their children and their children's children. They were selfless, so why are they the ones who have to suffer now? Why are they the ones that have to lose it all? Where is the fairness in that? I still don't know.

And then all thoughts fade away, into the background of my clouded brain, because I see *him.* The man who inspired me and whom I looked up to for years. The man who taught me everything I know, minute as it is, about construction and handy work. There he sits in one of the many worn and tattered chairs. Gazing straight ahead at the television in front of him, but not hearing a word of it.

Then before I know it I am looking at his grey-blue eyes hidden behind square glasses, snow-white hair, chin unshaven with stubble, ears that are too big, and a heartfelt smile spread across his worn and weathered face. Extra-large t-shirts, white undershirts, sweatpants, and black crocks messily draped on his body. Skin dry and forgotten, lips chapped and cracking, fingernails yellowy and uncut. But who stares back? The man I have known and loved for eighteen years of my life? No. A man who is a shadow of his former self stares back. Empty emotionless eyes swimming with question, searching for answers. *Who is this person looking at me? I have seen their face before, I have heard their voice, but why don't I know their name or how I know them? Why don't I know how they know me?*

"Hi PopPop. It's me . . ." I say gazing into the eyes of a man robbed of everything precious to him. A man wiped of memories. A man consumed by Alzheimer's. My hero, my PopPop taken away from me by Alzheimer's . . .

As Danielle so movingly illustrates, coping with a loved one's diagnosis is a traumatic experience. The grief that accompanies seeing your loved one become more like a stranger may be overwhelming. This grief may be experienced as a mental, physical, emotional, or social reaction and may include feelings of denial, anger, guilt, anxiety, sadness, and despair. Alzheimer's disease is a particularly difficult disease to cope with, in part because of the sadness inherent in seeing your loved one's mind deteriorate. This deterioration of the mind is why some people fear an Alzheimer's diagnosis even more than a cancer diagnosis. As legendary college basketball coach Jim Valvano said at the end of a famous speech in 1993, 10 years after being diagnosed with cancer, "Cancer can take away all of my physical ability. It cannot touch my mind; it cannot touch my heart; and it cannot touch my soul. And those three things are going to carry on forever."[24]

Before we explore the settings in which dementia care occurs, let's review the primary "reality lessons" learned about the illness of dementia and how to translate those lessons into both practical and realistic strategies.

LESSON 1: MUCH ABOUT DEMENTIA IS POORLY UNDERSTOOD

Strategies

1. While the scientific researchers and academicians continue to sort out the pieces of the dementia puzzle, your quality of life and that of your loved one are more likely to improve by *knowing the key issues in dementia that impact daily lives*. Reflecting on topics like driving, insight, anger, and delusions is a better use of your time than fretting about the relative contribution of vascular disease, Lewy bodies, and plaques and tangles to your loved one's illness.
2. *Don't get overly excited about preliminary findings in dementia research.* A good example of this is the debate over whether statins (drugs like atorvastatin [Lipitor] and rosuvastatin [Crestor] that lower cholesterol) prevent Alzheimer's

disease or other dementias. In November 2000, a study published in the journal *Lancet* found that individuals over the age of 50 who were prescribed statins had a substantially lowered risk of developing dementia.[25] A second study published in 2004 using the same case-control study design found that statin users had a 39 percent lower risk of Alzheimer's disease compared with nonstatin users.[26] Subsequently, however, two larger studies involving over 26,000 participants that were both double-blind, randomized, placebo-controlled trials showed no difference in the incidence of dementia between subjects who got a statin versus those who got a placebo.[27] We therefore now have good evidence to conclude that statins have little to no effect in preventing Alzheimer's or other dementias.

LESSON 2: TRUTH UNDERLIES MANY OF THE OVERUSED PHRASES ABOUT DEMENTIA

Strategy

Consider the following phrases, both of which I have heard many times since I completed my training in 1996:

1. *"If you've met one person with Alzheimer's, you've met one person with Alzheimer's."*

   This of course refers on one level to the fact that everyone with Alzheimer's disease remains a unique individual and deserves to be treated as an individual, not as a "disease." But it also refers to the fact that Alzheimer's is such an unpredictable, poorly understood disease that it really does differ tremendously in its manifestations from one person to another. Even when we try our best to use terms like "mild," "moderate," and "severe," or to use MMSE scores to discuss patients with colleagues, it's never possible to paint a true picture of a person with dementia. Quoting again from Jennifer Ghent-Fuller:

   Individuals are unique in their prior history, beliefs, behaviours and habits. Alzheimer disease progresses at different rates in different people: some succumb to it in as little as two years; others deteriorate slowly over twenty years. The changes that the person experiences at any one time depend on the area of the brain that have been affected. So, for example, some people develop language changes early in their illness, others maintain their fluency for years.[28]

2. *"She has good days and bad days."*

   This is one of those phrases that strike at the heart of the unpredictability of dementia. The typical explanations include familiarity of tasks and surroundings, overstimulation or understimulation, and stress and fatigue toward the end of the day. But I've heard family members insist that even when none of these conditions have occurred, there are significant differences observed day to day. In a July 2009 paper entitled (aptly) "Good Days and Bad Days in Dementia: A Qualitative Analysis of Variability in Symptom Expression," the authors analyzed what characteristics patients and caregivers describe as indicative of good days or bad days. Although it was a relatively small study (involving 31 community-dwelling people with dementia), it shed some light on this issue. A good day might be described as a day when the person has more interest in things or less agitation, while a bad day might include more verbal repetition or the occurrence of a single event that made the day bad. Good days were associated with increased initiation, better mood, and improved concentration, while bad days were associated with worse verbal repetition, anger, irritability, forgetfulness, delusions, and worsening mood.[29]

Lesson 3: Seek Out Early Recognition of Dementia

Strategies

1. Oppose the status quo. It's all too easy to rationalize that because there is no cure or highly effective treatment yet available, why bother seeking early recognition and diagnosis. But in fact that nihilistic view is now being challenged on a regular basis. Noting that patients with undiagnosed dementia typically go from crisis to crisis, with frequent visits to the emergency department and extensive testing, Dr. McCarten (quoted earlier in the chapter) notes that:

Through early diagnosis and proper chronic disease management, we hope to prevent this type of approach to care and put an end to the so-called pop-drop, where dad (or mom) is regularly brought to the emergency department because the family doesn't know what else to do. This type of acute care approach is expensive, ineffective, and grueling for patients and families.[30]

2. Realize that how Alzheimer's disease is diagnosed is rapidly changing. There is a growing consensus that the amyloid plaques that are characteristic of Alzheimer's disease actually begin accumulating in the brain decades before symptoms like memory loss and personality changes begin to display themselves. If Alzheimer's disease is viewed as a disease with a lengthy (years or decades) preclinical phase, the new goal is to identify people at risk of developing the clinical phase of Alzheimer's disease in the future so that drugs that can slow, modify, or halt the disease's progression will have the most effect.

Lesson 4: Lifestyle Changes Are Key to Your Alzheimer's Risk

Strategies

1. At the 2011 International Conference on Alzheimer's Disease, a study was presented that showed that seven risk factors contribute to more than half of the nearly 36 million people with Alzheimer's disease worldwide and nearly 60 percent of the nearly 6 million cases of Alzheimer's disease in the United States. The most important of these was physical inactivity, followed by depression, smoking, high blood pressure in midlife, obesity in midlife, low educational attainment, and diabetes.

2. Since there are presently no cures or treatments that modify the course of Alzheimer's disease, it's that much more important to concentrate on these preventive efforts. As Dr. Ronald Petersen, MD, PhD, professor of neurology and director of the Alzheimer's Disease Research Center at the Mayo Medical School put it after the study was published, "I think what we're realizing is that we can do something about this. We may not be able to prevent [Alzheimer's disease], or stop it in its tracks by lifestyle modification, but I think there are significant inroads that can be made into this disease."[31]

2

MY EXPERIENCE WITH ALZHEIMER'S DISEASE

In his recently published book *How We Age*, Marc Agronin, a fellow geriatric psychiatrist and friend, writes of the "risk that the retelling of a life, especially from the vantage point of a doctor, will not only fall short but will also end up trivializing certain aspects." He continues that "there is the greater risk that stories of medical or psychiatric ailments end up dehumanizing the patient, portraying him or her as a disease and not as a human being."[1]

When I read this, I couldn't help but realize that, for me, the motivation to devote my career to people with Alzheimer's disease (AD) and other dementias living in institutions was precisely to counter this dehumanization that is so rampant. Of all the disorders we are vulnerable to, none is more dehumanizing than Alzheimer's disease. What better way to counter the dehumanization, the stigma, and the despair that this disease causes than to teach people about it, to counter the myths, the biases, and the rush to judgment? After pointing out the irony of his "great communicator" father becoming aphasic (losing his language abilities) in the early years of his Alzheimer's disease, President Reagan's son Ron told CNN's Larry King in a recent Alzheimer's disease special that in some ways his father was lucky to escape "a lot of the worst symptoms, like anger and paranoia." As he put it, quite simply, "It's not the patient's fault if they begin behaving in odd ways."[2] Yet the reality is that many people, including health care professionals, continue to behave as if it is the patient's fault. By educating people and providing knowledge and alternative coping strategies, perhaps this will improve.

I believe a prevailing attitude among a generation of people is that because there's no cure for this disease that is already so feared and misunderstood, it's better to tune it out and pretend it doesn't exist. Actor Seth Rogan's fiancé Lauren Miller, whose mother was diagnosed with Alzheimer's disease at age 55, realizes the problem when she says (also on the Larry King special): "The things that make me angry are that unfortunately this disease gets very little attention, especially with people that are our age, they know very little about it."[3] Ronald Petersen, director of the Mayo Clinic Alzheimer's Disease Research Center, warned that "if we don't do something about Alzheimer's disease right now, Alzheimer's disease in and of itself may bankrupt the healthcare system."[4] It's truly amazing to me that people are tuning out a disease that is likely to affect 100 million people by 2050.

In 2007, I received a Teaching Recognition Award from the Warren Alpert Medical School of Brown University. This came about primarily as a result of my monthly teaching sessions with the Geriatric Medicine Fellows at Brown, sessions in which young doctors studying to be geriatricians brought their difficult cases and clinical challenges for me to comment on. As you'll see in Chapter 10, we have a real crisis on our hands when it comes to our health care workforce being attracted to geriatric work. Recommendations from studies that have suggested a need for 36,000 additional geriatricians by 2030 have been shot down as "impossible and unrealistic," in part because fewer than 320 physicians entered geriatric fellowship training programs from 2004 to 2008. I viewed my monthly sessions as an opportunity to keep these bright, hard-working doctors interested and excited about their work with the elderly. The way I saw it, I was the lucky one. These geriatric fellows were dealing with managing not only the dementia-related mood and behavior problems of their patients, but also the heart problems, high blood pressure, diabetes, and arthritis. To me, nothing could be more fascinating and intellectually stimulating than talking about someone who sees members of a local symphony orchestra coming into his dining room on a nightly basis to perform, or someone who believes his spouse has been replaced with an imposter. Having received a master of public health degree in epidemiology along with my medical degree at the University of Michigan, I was convinced that only by reaching large numbers of people through teaching and sharing information could I make a significant impact on those affected by dementia.

To reach people, lecturing is one venue that I truly enjoy. At the 2011 Annual Meeting of the Rhode Island Assisted Living Association (RIALA), I gave a lecture about when having dementia necessitates secure living arrangements. To put it more simply, when is it time for someone to move to a locked unit? As you'll learn much more about in Chapter 5, a growing trend in assisted living is secure dementia units, that is, units with locked doors to prevent wandering and with (in theory at least) more educated staff and structured activities programs. I knew this lecture would be difficult and somewhat controversial, due in part to the many stakeholders and the emotional and financial factors involved. These units are typically more expensive, more stigmatized, and by their nature restrict freedom of residents. Rhode Island's Department of Health, for example, has been advocating for more and more residents with dementia, even in the mild stages, to be transferred to these secure units, arguing that issues of safety and potential wandering risks must trump all others. In the lecture, I tried to be balanced and informed about the issues, yet open to a sharing of ideas and disagreements. In my view, these are the elements of a successful lecture. Fortunately, I somehow managed to succeed, as I received this thank you from the organization's executive director:

Hi Dr. Andy,

Thank you so much for sharing your expertise on dementia at our annual conference. As always people loved your session . . . so informative and thought provoking. I know how busy you are and want you to know how much we appreciate the time you generously share with us. As you know the Department of Health is giving us a run for our money on care of people with dementia. We are making progress but it is slow and uphill all the way.

We had a great turnout for the conference and people raved about the breakout sessions . . . terrific is the word we heard most often. Thank you doesn't seem to convey how much we appreciate your support of RIALA. I hope you understand how much we appreciate all you do. If I can ever be of any assistance to you, please do not hesitate to contact me.

Sincerely,
Kathleen

I'll close this chapter with a case I had recently that illustrates many of the themes and concepts explored in this book. It was only after treating many patients like these in many settings that I realized I had something unique to offer to people as they meet their own dementia-related situations.

M. C. is an 89-year-old woman admitted to an assisted living facility after her two daughters, clearly at their wits' end, brought her there under the false pretense of going out to lunch with them at a local restaurant. She had a seven-year history of slowly progressive memory decline and had been treated with donepezil (Aricept) for the past five years. She had divorced her first husband after only two years of marriage and was a widow after her second husband (of 35 years) died. She had been a fiercely independent and strong-willed person who had worked as a hospital payroll clerk. She had no history of smoking or drinking and had never had any psychiatric problems warranting treatment. Her overall health was quite good: she had a history of diverticulitis, osteopenia, hypertension, and a thyroid goiter. She was taking few medications, only a baby aspirin and the blood pressure medicine lisinopril (Zestril) in addition to the Aricept.

Shortly after admission to the assisted living facility, she wrote an emotional letter to her daughters, arguing vehemently that she was "perfectly capable of managing my own affairs." Over the next several weeks, she developed increasing anger, paranoia, and agitation, culminating in a four-day hunger strike and threats to "jump out the window." When I saw her for my first visit, I found her to be intelligent and engaging. She was slightly anxious but showed no signs of disabling anxiety, depression, or paranoia. She was well oriented and attentive but clearly had significant problems with short-term memory and other aspects of cognition. Her insight was poor, as she underestimated her deficits and exhibited poor judgment. For example, she insisted she was perfectly capable of taking her medications on her own, yet she had difficulty recalling what those medications even were. She spoke disparagingly of her daughters, in particular one that "wants to be in total control of me." On a brief dementia screening test, she scored 18 out of 30, indicating a moderate degree of dementia. Her daughters had recounted multiple instances when she had been scammed and taken advantage of financially, along with many car accidents and episodes of getting lost. Chapter 9 is an in-depth discussion of issues concerning mental capacity and decision making in dementia, with a special emphasis on financial capacity.

She refused my suggestion of taking a new medication, and because of the ensuing hunger strike and threats to kill herself, she was hospitalized in a geriatric psychiatry inpatient unit shortly thereafter. As you will learn in Chapter 7, the psychiatry inpatient unit is an important aspect of dementia care that more and more people are coming in contact with. It has its strengths and weaknesses, but certainly one of its strengths is the provision of convenient high-level specialized assessments as well as 24-hour monitoring and supervision that is sometimes essential to treat urgent problems quickly. For M. C., this meant obtaining detailed neuropsychological testing, testing that can not only confirm a diagnosis of Alzheimer's disease but also point out relative strengths and weaknesses that may help staff and family improve the person's quality of life. In M. C.'s case, this testing revealed moderate to severe deficits in language, recall, visuospatial abilities, new learning, and executive functioning. In Alzheimer's disease, visuospatial problems may cause an individual to become disoriented or lost in familiar environments, and the ability to recognize familiar individuals may become impaired. Executive functioning includes the ability to plan projects, formulate goals and objectives, prioritize, apply self-discipline, and remember steps involved in complex tasks. Alzheimer's disease deteriorates executive functioning so that it becomes increasingly difficult for an individual to carry out daily tasks and live independently.

An occupational therapist trained in doing functional assessments of people with memory loss provided another useful type of test while M. C. was in the hospital. This test showed that M.C. had a great deal of difficulty with issues involving safety, medication administration, money management, and meal preparation and planning.

Of these, medication management is especially critical. Helping your loved one with Alzheimer's disease take his or her medications safely is one of the more important aspects of Alzheimer's caregiving. Medication errors are the most common type of error made in health care, and the Institute of Medicine estimates that 1.5 million preventable adverse drug events occur annually in the United States. While proper, prudent use of medications may help to maintain your loved one's quality of life and avoid unnecessary hospitalizations and medical problems, the opposite may occur when medications are used improperly or unsafely. Too often, doctors may assume you have a system to give medications and an understanding of side effects, when in fact you may not. In M. C.'s case, the problem of medication administration was even harder because of her insistence that she didn't need anyone's help to take her medications properly.

After a 10-day hospital stay, M. C. returned to the assisted living facility, on the antipsychotic medication olanzapine (Zyprexa) and a low dose of the antianxiety medication lorazepam (Ativan). She also had her thyroid status evaluated while in the hospital and was placed on the thyroid medication propylthiouracil (PTU). Her behavior improved considerably, she became more social and involved in activities, and she was no longer paranoid about her daughter. She was still angry with her daughter but admitted she "never should have starved myself." She even told me she felt "much better since my brain started working right."

By sharing this case and in fact this book, I hope to convey a sense of optimism that even though we do not currently have a cure and dementia presents tremendous challenges, there is no doubt in my mind that for the vast majority of patients and their caregivers, an improved quality of life is attainable.

3

CAREGIVERS, COSTS, AND CONCERNS

At its very core, the reality of Alzheimer's disease (AD) is that the caregiver often suffers more than the person with the disease. For one thing, how can overwhelmed caregivers possibly understand and benefit from the suggestions in this book about nursing homes, assisted living facilities, memory clinics, and hospitals if they don't have some strategies to help themselves? And how can caregivers struggling with recession, unemployment, and other financial burdens possibly navigate through the maze of insurance, government programs, and personal assets to actually pay for their loved ones' care? While some of this information is included in individual chapters, I'll try to consolidate the important caregiver-related issues here. The related topic of respite care is addressed in detail in Chapter 6.

CAREGIVER HEALTH

Amazingly, it's been only in the past few years that the importance of the health of the dementia caregiver has been recognized and appreciated. It of course makes perfect sense that only with a healthy and involved caregiver can a person with dementia have optimal treatment and quality of life. Wouldn't it be nice if physicians and other health care providers viewed caregivers as allies and partners as opposed to "problems" or impediments to the care of their loved ones?

This tension has several explanations and root causes. For one thing, the mere fact that the caregiver is having an interaction with the provider usually implies there is a problem: there aren't many "well visits" when it comes to dementia. So the caregiver is looking for help, for suggestions, for answers, and this requires time, effort, thought, and even experience that often the provider just doesn't have. Second, the whole concept of the doctor-patient relationship is potentially disrupted by the presence of the caregiver. What is the best way for this communication to occur? My goal here is to provide caregivers with some useful strategies to appropriately work with their loved ones' health care providers toward the common goal of improving their loved ones' quality of life.

The scope of the problem is staggering: nearly 15 million Americans are now providing care for someone with Alzheimer's disease or another type of dementia, with increasing numbers expected. These caregivers provide billions of hours of unpaid care that is valued at more than $202 billion annually and that contributes to the physical, emotional, and financial burdens faced by caregivers on a regular basis. Higher rates of depression and anxiety as well as poorer health and self-care habits are only a few of the many problems faced by dementia caregivers. Compared with those who are not caregivers, dementia caregivers have been found to have higher levels of stress hormones, reduced immune function, slower wound healing, and more heart disease and high blood pressure.[1]

Dementia caregiving is so stressful that it may even lead to higher rates of dementia in the caregiving spouse, as was found in one recent study. This study was not a small, insignificant study published in an obscure journal. Rather, published in the well-regarded *Journal of the American Geriatrics Society*, it looked at 1,221 married couples without dementia age 65 years and older from Utah who were studied for up to 12 years to monitor for dementia onset in husbands, wives, or both. Over those 12 years, 125 cases of dementia in the husband only were diagnosed, 70 cases in the wife only, and 30 cases in both spouses. Having a spouse with dementia was associated with a six-fold increased risk of developing dementia. While the authors acknowledged that the reasons for the increased risk are not clear, the results suggest that having a spouse with dementia is a risk factor for the nondemented spouse developing dementia.[2] Why might that be? Well, for one thing, the practical burden of caregiving combined with the stoicism that many spouses have is a recipe for disaster: stress levels rise, eating and exercise habits plummet, opportunities for hobbies and socialization vanish, and levels of depression skyrocket.

INFLUENCE OF STRESS ON MEMORY

How stress may contribute to dementia warrants some explanation. Stress is a normal response to threatening or dangerous events. Our stress response (also called the fight-or-flight response) can give us a jolt of energy, strength, focus, and alertness to help in emergencies. But when stress becomes chronic, it stops being helpful and leads to adverse effects on our bodies, minds, and emotions. The brain is an excellent example of how chronic stress leads to problems with learning and memory.

On a chemical level, low to moderate levels of stress hormones like cortisol and adrenaline can improve memory, while higher levels seem to disrupt memory. Stressors can produce lapses in attention, and it may take longer to make decisions. If you're not able to concentrate on a subject in the first place, you won't remember it later. With chronic stress, hormones that turn on the fight-or-flight response, like adrenaline, may remain active in your brain too long. This may eventually injure and even kill cells in the hippocampus, a brain area critical for memory and learning. Interestingly, it is the hippocampus that is affected early on in Alzheimer's disease.

High levels of cortisol due to chronic stress seem to induce depression as well. The connection between depression and memory loss has been known for years, with a leading theory being that during periods of stress, the high levels of cortisol that are produced cause damage to connections between brain cells. In fact, Dr. George Alexopolous, a psychiatry professor at Cornell University, told the *Wall Street Journal* that "depression creates a tremendous burden to a brain that already had increased predisposition to dementia."[3] People with low levels of stress in their lives are likely better able to tolerate age-related brain changes.

It is unrealistic to eliminate all stress from your life. Rather, the key is managing stress so that it doesn't spiral out of control and affect your functioning. I've listed several key strategies for managing stress at the conclusion of this chapter.

COMMUNICATION STRATEGIES

One of the most prominent sources of stress that dementia caregivers tell me they have is that of trying to communicate with their loved ones. Let's explore this issue of communication in more detail. Although we often take it for granted, communication is what connects us to each other. Unfortunately, dementia creates barriers to communication that strain our relationships with our loved ones. Communication is a verbal or nonverbal way of relating to another, and the good news is that people with Alzheimer's disease often maintain their nonverbal communication skills until very late in the course of their illness. Verbal skills, on the other hand, deteriorate much earlier and have to be given less and less importance by caregivers if they wish to preserve their sanity. Examples of problems with verbal abilities in Alzheimer's disease include trouble finding the correct words, repeating words and phrases, and creating new words for ones that are forgotten. Patience and reassurance are both critical when it comes to communication. If your loved one is having trouble communicating, reassure him or her and explain that you'll do your best to try to understand what he or she means. Although this is much easier said than done, try to avoid correcting or criticizing speech problems that you observe. Remembering "the 3 Rs" is useful: repeat, reassure, and redirect. Redirection is especially helpful: if your loved one is having difficulty or getting agitated with a certain activity, redirect him to a less stressful task. Sometimes just bringing up a favorite topic or memory will do the trick, as may providing a favorite object to focus on.

Keep telling yourself that nonverbal communication offers the best chance for success. While the content of your loved one's message may be hard to understand, it's often possible to uncover the feelings behind it by observing tone of voice, facial expressions, gestures, and body language. Speaking clearly in a relaxed tone of voice will put your loved one at ease. Friendly gestures also foster positive interactions.

COPING WITH THE GRIEF OF DIAGNOSIS

How does a caregiver possibly cope with the grief of a loved one's diagnosis of Alzheimer's disease? Imagine how hard it is to see your loved one becoming more and more like a stranger over time. Many caregivers have told me how they grieve twice: when Alzheimer's starts and again at death. This "anticipatory grief" is an emotional pain that's felt long before the person actually dies. It may rise with periods of more rapid mental or physical decline and fall again when things temporarily stabilize. What makes Alzheimer's disease especially difficult to cope with is of course seeing your loved one's mind deteriorate. This may be why many people fear an Alzheimer's diagnosis even more than a cancer diagnosis.

Everyone grieves differently, and grief may include feelings of denial, anger, guilt, anxiety, sadness, and despair. How you grieve will depend in part on your relationship with your loved one, your own coping skills, and support you receive from others. Occasions like birthdays, holidays, and anniversaries are especially tough, perhaps because you see your loved one contributing less and less to the life of the family. Caregiver support groups may be particularly helpful in these scenarios since friends and family members may not understand how you can be grieving while the person you're caring for is still alive.

WHAT REALLY HAPPENS AT A CAREGIVER SUPPORT GROUP?

I must admit that didn't really know what to expect when I led my first caregiver support group. It was at a long-term care facility that had residents in all stages of Alzheimer's disease, from people with early, mild disease living independently in apartments to those with severe dementia receive total care in the nursing home section of the building.

I had been told only that several family members had requested that the facility run a support group to help them cope with their loved one's illness as well as learn more about dementia and what treatments could help. With little formal training in group dynamics or facilitation of a therapy group, I found myself in mostly unchartered territory. Yet I believe my having few preconceived notions helped the participants achieve their goals.

There was a core group of about 15 family members that met monthly for evening sessions, and we eventually had about 10 sessions. There were daughters, sons, daughters-in-law, siblings, and even close friends. The emotions displayed were powerful and at times disconcerting. I recall one daughter who had extreme disbelief at what was happening to her mother and refused to accept the reality of her mother's illness. One family marveled at the patience of the nurses and aides, while another complained bitterly about the lack of substantive activities. A spouse whose husband with dementia had recently died channeled all of her energies into understanding the details of her husband's brain autopsy: Did he truly have Alzheimer's disease or was it a different type of dementia? The most challenging participants were those who wanted to monopolize the session to challenge or second-guess the medications that their loved one's physician had chosen, but fortunately other group members intervened when that got out of hand.

Most wanted what you would probably guess: information and education, strategies for better communicating with their loved ones, and reassurance that their approach and ideas were in sync with others.

While I enjoyed my role in these sessions as teacher and educator, I think the most benefit came from giving the group members permission to say what was on their minds despite feelings of shame, anger, frustration, embarrassment, or inadequacy. The comfort level that developed after a few sessions was invaluable at fostering helpful discussions, and certain themes tended to come up time and again. One session we spent nearly the entire 90 minutes on two questions: Is it ok to take mom out for a family wedding even if she will take 3 days to recover from the agitation she will inevitably experience after returning? and What should I do about my brother who refuses to visit mom because he can't handle seeing her like this?

WHO ARE THE CAREGIVERS?

After a number of years of leading caregiver support groups and delivering lectures on dementia, I realized that often I was speaking to a room with a female to male ratio of 9:1. Somewhat surprisingly, then, I found that according to the 2011 Alzheimer's Disease Facts and Figures report issued by the Alzheimer's Association, 60 percent of family caregivers and other unpaid caregivers of people with AD and other dementias are women. I would've guessed much higher.

Most caregivers are age 55 years or older, and nearly half have either full- or part-time jobs. Half of all unpaid caregivers live in the same household as the person receiving the care, and a quarter have children younger than age 18 living with them. Many caregivers, usually in their thirties or forties, are often called the sandwich generation because they provide care for two generations at the same time. Believe it or not, there is even a group referred to as the club sandwich generation. This refers to a generation that is helping to care for three other

generations. Usually members of the club sandwich generation are caring for elderly parents, providing some support for adult children and helping to care for
grandchildren. With couples having children later in life and some individuals
starting second families after divorce or the death or a spouse, some members of
the club sandwich generation may still have young children in the home.

Many caregivers of people with dementia make major changes to their work
schedules because of the stresses and responsibilities of caregiving. According
to the Alzheimer's Association, two-thirds said they had to go in late, leave
early, or take time off, and 20 percent had to take a leave of absence. Imagine
the countless numbers of stressed and sleep-deprived dementia caregivers
who go to work distracted, anxious about what the next phone call might be,
and otherwise unable to devote their intellectual resources to their work. This
idea of "presenteeism" is especially relevant in these situations: caregivers may
be physically present at work, but because they are absorbed in the task of caregiving, they are mentally absent. The sheer number of phone calls caregivers
receive can be mind-boggling: forgetfulness and anxiety alone can lead to
mom calling her daughter 10 times during the day at work, then another five
or six times during the night.

Dementia caregivers are different from other caregivers. Practically, they provide more help with personal care, such as providing help with getting in and
out of bed, and getting to and from the toilet. Emotionally, the close relationship
they have with their loved ones makes it especially hard; the years or even decades of shared emotions, memories, and experiences can't be just put aside.

Dementia caregivers are also more likely to advocate for their loved ones
with government agencies and other providers, and to supervise care in the
community. Because they are so involved with their loved one with dementia,
they often spend less time with their families than other caregivers, and they
experience more physical, emotional, and financial strain than other caregivers.
All of these factors combine to put the dementia caregiver at especially high risk
of caregiver burnout, a phenomenon that usually refers to overwhelming anger,
irritability, anxiety, fatigue, and sleep problems.

SUPPORT FOR DEMENTIA CAREGIVERS

Fortunately, caregivers are beginning to get the attention they deserve. For
one thing, doctors and other health care professionals are realizing that caregivers are often the key to treating the person with dementia. By finding sources
of help for caregiver tasks, providing support for caregivers, and monitoring for
symptoms of depression in caregivers, doctors are actually treating their
patients with dementia with some of the most effective tools available.

For the first time, researchers are even developing models of caregiver support. For example, the Savvy Caregiver Program, developed at the University
of Minnesota, builds caregivers' knowledge, skills, and self-confidence. It is an
evidence-based dementia care training program that has been designated as

one of the approved dementia training programs of the Alzheimer's Disease Demonstration Grants to States program, funded through the U.S. Administration on Aging. The Savvy Caregiver DVD was completed in 2007 and released to the public in January 2008. The four-DVD set sells for $49.95, and there is even an optional homework CD-ROM that asks caregivers to complete a homework assignment for each of the four DVDs.[4]

Begun in 1995, the Resources for Enhancing Alzheimer's Caregiver Health (REACH) initiative has as its primary purpose finding ways to teach caregivers how to handle difficult behaviors, how to manage their own stress levels, and how to maintain their social supports. Funded by the National Institutes of Health, it involves research from six universities.[5]

The primary elements of successful interventions for dementia caregivers are education, support, and counseling, along with various combinations of these strategies. Education, for example, may include reading books like this, exploring high-quality Internet sites on dementia, attending lectures and discussions, and even developing new skills to respond to particular behaviors and situations that may emerge. Support groups are ideal when they provide a comfortable, nonthreatening atmosphere that lends itself to openly discussing feelings, attitudes, successes, and failures of dementia care. Exchanging ideas and learning from others are essential. Finally, counseling involves a relationship between the caregiver and a trained therapy professional. Helping to cope with stresses, manage emotions and time management, and develop problem-solving abilities are only a few of the possibilities of counseling or psychotherapy.

Costs of Dementia Caregiving

The realities of caring for a person with dementia are sobering. Just when a caregiver has figured out how to handle his or her loved one's personality changes and communication limitations, she wakes up realizing she has to now tackle the burden of paying for this care. No one is spared the financial pain when it comes to dementia. Caregivers cost their employers an estimated $36.5 billion a year in lost productivity, missed work, and hiring replacement workers. Caregivers may refuse promotions, and many come to work but are unable to perform their jobs well because of the overwhelming stress of caregiving. Businesses spend another $24.6 billion annually on health and long-term care costs for employees with dementia. With people working later in life and delaying retirement because of the recession and other issues, more and more people with early onset and mild dementia are still working.

Sibling Disputes

An increasingly familiar scenario is that described by LuMarie Polivka-West in an August 2011 newspaper article entitled "Housing bust Impedes Move to

Assisted Living." When her mother, an 86-year-old retired nurse with Alzheimer's disease, started wandering from her Florida home in 2007, Polivka-West started planning to move her parents (including her 94-year-old father) to assisted living. But because of the collapse in the real estate market, she couldn't sell her parents' house, and she and her two brothers had to each contribute $600 per month to afford the $3,200 per month assisted living apartment. To me, the most telling aspect of Polivka-West's story was her quote that although "it was a significant cost to me and my brothers," they didn't let their parents know about the financial issues. Referring to her parents, she states that "it didn't cause them anxiety, just us."[6]

This pressure on families to pay for their parents' and grandparents' placements, or to take over the care themselves, has added another reason for sibling disputes related to Alzheimer's disease. I've seen siblings fight over virtually everything related to Alzheimer's disease, including how bad off their loved one really is, where their loved one should be living, and who should be paying for their care. Two or three sibs may "gang up" on the one who has power of attorney and accuse her of poor communication, being a "control freak," or even isolating their loved one with dementia.

WHO PAYS FOR DEMENTIA CARE?

Alzheimer's disease easily triples health care costs for those over the age of 65. The average family caregiver for someone age 50 years or older spent $5,531 annually on caregiving expenses in 2007. Incontinence supplies alone can cost up to $1,800 per year. Medicaid costs are over 9 times higher for Alzheimer's care, as people with Alzheimer's disease consume extraordinary amounts of hospital care, long-term care, and care for comorbid medical problems like heart disease and diabetes.

In part because of our chaotic and complicated health care system, most people are poorly informed about who pays for Alzheimer's care. For example, many people mistakenly believe Medicare covers long-term care, and few purchase long-term care insurance. Only 10 percent of the elderly have private long-term care insurance (nearly 25 percent of people who apply for long-term care insurance are declined coverage because of health issues), and the limited nature of these plans means that only 4 percent of long-term care expenditures are paid by private insurance, while 33 percent of expenditures are paid out of pocket. In addition, having a diagnosis of Alzheimer's disease or other type of dementia will likely lead to rejection of your long-term care insurance policy application, so think about coverage at a younger age if possible. Policies vary greatly, so read the fine print. These policies are designed to cover the costs of a nursing home or assisted living facility. Nursing home costs for an individual with Alzheimer's disease range from $42,000 to more than $72,000 per year, which is clearly unaffordable for most families. Assisted living facilities are somewhat less expensive: average costs for a one-bedroom unit are in the range of $2,800 per month, and about a third of facilities charge a one-time entrance fee.

One aspect of President Obama's new health care reform law offers help in caring for people with dementia. This provision, the Community Living Assistance Services and Supports (CLASS) Act, would be funded by premiums and would pay enrollees $50 or more per day if they became too disabled to perform normal daily activities like eating and bathing. Employers who choose to participate would sign up their employees, who would then have the ability to opt out. The cash benefits could be applied to nursing home care, but in an effort to encourage enrollees to stay in their own homes, payouts could cover such things as wheelchair ramps and wages for home health care aides. But CLASS Act benefits aren't expected to begin flowing until 2018, and the program has already generated a lot of controversy related to its fiscal implications.[7] In fact, in early February 2012, the CLASS Act was officially repealed by the House of Representatives. For it to be fully annulled, the Senate must also vote in favor of doing away with it, and the president must sign off on the repeal.

You might think that disability insurance makes sense to pay for Alzheimer's care, but as with long-term care insurance, you need to have the policy before a diagnosis is made. Now that there is a new category for diagnosing Alzheimer's disease in a preclinical phase that may start decades before symptoms appear, it remains to be seen whether a person diagnosed with preclinical Alzheimer's disease needs to have a disability policy in place prior to receiving that diagnosis. Even if you're lucky enough to have a prior disability policy in place when you develop Alzheimer's disease, chances are good that it will only pay one-half to two-thirds of your salary if you're unable to work.

Since 48 million Americans are currently enrolled in the Medicare insurance program, let's look at what Medicare really does cover. Medicare is a federal program that provides government-funded insurance coverage to people age 65 years or older and people with certain disabilities. Typically, Medicare covers 80 percent of nonhospital costs and 100 percent of inpatient hospital costs after the patient meets a deductible. Under certain limited conditions, Medicare will pay some nursing home costs for beneficiaries who require skilled nursing or rehabilitation services. To be covered, you must receive the services from a Medicare-certified skilled nursing home after a qualifying hospital stay. A qualifying hospital stay is the amount of time spent in a hospital just prior to entering a nursing home, which must be at least three days.

For Medicare beneficiaries receiving outpatient mental health treatment, which includes people living in assisted living facilities and nursing homes, Medicare has had a longstanding discriminatory practice of covering only 50 percent of costs. As an example, consider a nursing home resident with mild Alzheimer's disease who is still quite functional, dressing and bathing herself with only minimal assistance but who is unable to live at home or in an assisted living facility because of her severe chronic obstructive pulmonary disease (COPD) and medication needs. She is depressed and highly anxious, with

regular panic attacks that cause her heart to race and her to be terrified that she
will collapse with a heart attack. If she is already my patient and I am asked to
see her for a follow-up psychiatric visit, the Medicare payment I receive (and
the copayment she will be billed for) will differ depending on what my diagnosis
is for that visit. If I diagnose her with Panic Disorder, her copay will be significantly higher than if my diagnosis were Dementia due to Alzheimer's Disease,
with Depressed Mood, because a dementia diagnosis is usually not subject to
the "outpatient psychiatric limitation."

Before the Medicare Improvements for Patients and Providers Act (MIPPA)
was signed into law on July 15, 2008, patients paid half the cost of Medicare-
covered outpatient mental health services, but only 20 percent of the cost of
Medicare-covered outpatient medical services. MIPPA equalized the coverage
rates so that as of January 1, 2014, Medicare Part B will pay outpatient mental
health services at the same level as other Part B services. The change to full par-
ity is gradual, so every year Medicare pays a certain percentage more than
50 percent (according to a formula) until 80 percent is reached in 2014.

The phase-in process and percentages apply to claims for professional services provided by physicians, clinical psychologists, clinical social workers, nurse
practitioners, clinical nurse specialists, and physician assistants. The phase-in
process also applies to diagnostic psychological and neuropsychological testing
to evaluate a patient's progress during treatment. As you might guess, these
services are highly relevant to people with dementia since much of dementia
treatment targets the behavioral and psychological symptoms that accompany
the illness.

Other initiatives are in the works to boost Medicare coverage for people with
Alzheimer's disease. The most important of these is probably the Health Outcomes, Planning, and Education (HOPE) for Alzheimer's Act, which is one of
the Alzheimer's Association's top federal priorities for the 112th Congress.
The HOPE for Alzheimer's Act would:

- Provide Medicare coverage for a package of services, including clinical diagnosis of Alzheimer's disease and care planning to provide those with the disease
  and their caregivers information about medical and nonmedical options for
  treatment and support services
- Require documentation of the diagnostic evaluation and any care planning
  provided in an individual's primary medical record[8]

Medicare Supplemental Insurance, often called Medigap because it helps pay
for gaps in Medicare coverage such as deductibles and coinsurances, is secon-
dary insurance that is sold by private health insurance companies nationwide.
Federal and state laws outline what Medigap policies are required to cover,
and some plans offer more extensive coverage than others.

Medicaid is a state and federal program that pays most nursing home costs for
people with limited incomes and assets. Eligibility varies by state, so you need to

check your state's requirements to learn if you are eligible. Medicaid will pay only for nursing home care provided in a facility certified by the government to provide service to Medicaid recipients. Practically, this means that millions of Americans who need nursing home care but can't afford to pay for it have to "spend down" their assets, become poor enough to qualify for Medicaid, and then move to nursing homes that the program covers. The rules for Medicaid are complicated and change often. There are income and asset limits for eligibility. For couples, if one person needs nursing home care, the spouse in the nursing home may be eligible for Medicaid and the spouse in the community can still keep enough assets and income to prevent impoverishment.

For those who are eligible, Medicaid covers most costs related to nursing home care. Medicaid pays for room and meals, the nursing home staff, nurses, therapists, doctor's visits, some prescription drugs, dental care, medical equipment such as wheelchairs, eyeglasses, and hearing aids. Medicaid does not pay for podiatrists, chiropractors, naturopaths, and independent providers such as psychologists, speech pathologists, audiologists, and physical therapists unless these services occur in a clinic setting. Medicaid usually does not pay for a single room and does not pay for televisions or phones.

Under federal law, nursing facilities must inform each resident who is entitled to Medicaid benefits (in writing, at the time of admission to the facility or when the resident becomes eligible for Medicaid) of the items and services that are included in nursing facility services under Medicaid. The facility must also give notice to residents about other items and services that the facility offers and which of these are not covered by Medicaid and for which the resident may be charged, including the amount of charges for those services. This information must be provided whenever changes in the charges go into effect.

Social Security is responsible for two major programs that provide benefits based on disability: Social Security Disability Insurance (SSDI), which is based on prior work under Social Security, and Supplemental Security Income (SSI). Under SSI, payments are made on the basis of financial need.

Social Security Disability Insurance (SSDI) is financed with Social Security taxes paid by employees, employers, and self-employed persons. To be eligible for a Social Security benefit and to be "insured" for Social Security purposes, the worker must earn sufficient credits based on taxable work. Disability benefits are payable to workers who are blind or disabled, widow(er)s, and adults who have been disabled since childhood. The amount of the monthly disability benefit is based on the Social Security earnings record of the insured worker. SSDI is a significant benefit for individuals with early onset Alzheimer's disease since these individuals are usually younger than 65 and often unable to work. In addition to a monthly payment, it serves as entry to Medicare benefits for those under the age of 65. Family members (e.g., spouses and minor children) may also be eligible for benefits based on the applicant's work record.

Supplemental Security Income (SSI) is a program financed through general revenues. SSI benefits are paid each month to individuals who have limited income and resources (assets) and are elderly or blind, or who have disabilities. The "disability" criteria for SSI are the same as for SSDI benefits. Unlike SSDI, eligibility for SSI is not based on prior work experience. In addition, in most states, individuals who receive SSI are also automatically eligible for Medicaid benefits.

Generally, if you enter a nursing home or hospital (or other medical facility) where Medicaid pays for more than half of the cost of your care, your SSI benefit is limited to $30 a month. Some states supplement this $30 benefit.

Under the Compassionate Allowance Initiative, the Social Security Administration (SSA) finds individuals with certain diseases and conditions eligible for Social Security Disability (SSDI) and Supplemental Security Income (SSI) benefits by the nature of the disease. While applicants still have to meet other SSDI criteria and/or SSI criteria, when it comes to the disability criterion, they are considered eligible by virtue of the disease and fast-tracked for a favorable decision about their eligibility for SSDI and SSI benefits. Fortunately, the Social Security Administration (SSA) has added early onset Alzheimer's to the list of conditions under its Compassionate Allowance Initiative, giving those with the disease expedited access to SSDI and SSI.

Other aspects of President Obama's health care reform law have particular relevance for people with Alzheimer's disease. They include the following:

- Establishment of an Innovation Center at the Centers for Medicare and Medicaid Services (CMS) to test various ways to promote care coordination in the Medicare program, with language specifically encouraging CMS to test care coordination models that include people with cognitive impairment and dementia
- Creation of an Independence at Home pilot project to provide high-cost Medicare beneficiaries, including those with Alzheimer's, with coordinated, primary care services in lower-cost settings, rather than more expensive institutional settings
- Permission for groups of health care providers who join together to provide care for Medicare patients to share in any cost-savings they would achieve by being more efficient and cost-effective, provided that these Accountable Care Organizations coordinate care for those with multiple chronic conditions

Before moving on to exploring the reality of dementia care in nursing homes, let's review the primary "reality lessons" learned about dementia caregivers and how to translate those lessons into practical, realistic strategies to maximize both the caregiver and the resident's quality of life.

Lesson 1: Tips for Managing Stress

Strategies

1. Identify the source of your caregiving stress and develop ways to tackle it head on.
2. Take better control of your reactions, thoughts, and emotions.

3. Take better care of yourself.
4. Make time for rest and relaxation.
5. Educate yourself about dementia and the stressful situations that it leads to.
6. Maintain or strengthen your network of supportive friends and family.
7. Fill your own prescriptions and keep your own doctor appointments.

Lesson 2: Work More Effectively with Your Loved One's Health Care Provider

Strategies

1. Develop confidence that you are a crucial part of your loved one's life and future. If you are meek and timid when it comes to your loved one's care, your own quality of life as well as your loved one's will likely suffer.
2. Devise appropriate, reasonable ways to be heard and understood by your loved one's health care team. While you may not want to think of yourself as a health care advocate, that's really what you are.
3. Acknowledge and assert yourself as a crucial part of the health care team. For example, the AD8 Dementia Screening Interview is an eight-item questionnaire that distinguishes between people who have dementia and those who don't. Two or more "yes" answers is strongly suggestive of dementia. In addition to its use as a screening test for Alzheimer's disease, the AD8 is especially useful to help you become involved as a caregiver. You complete the AD8 at home in the presence of your loved one and then bring the results to the next appointment. This not only may help the clinician more effectively treat your loved one, but it sends a strong message that you want and expect to be involved in his or her care. The AD8 may be downloaded at http://alzheimer .wustl.edu/About_Us/PDFs/AD8form2005.pdf
4. Keep track of important information. A written record of current medications and health problems, key contacts, appointments, and outcomes for each doctor visit may be helpful for all those involved in your loved one's care.

Lesson 3: Don't Panic about the Prospect of Paying for Your Loved One's Dementia Care

Strategies

1. As you've learned by reading this chapter, you're far from alone in having this situation to face. And because the landscape of options is complicated, it's imperative to keep your wits about you. Organizing and decluttering your financial documents is essential, as is holding an in-person or virtual meeting with family members and others with a vested interest in your loved one's future. A financial advisor may be helpful, but before that be sure to gather essential documents such as bank statements, insurance policies, unpaid bills, and credit card and mortgage statements.

2. Develop confidence that you can tackle this challenge. Just as you need to be confident in being a health care advocate, you need similar confidence in the financial aspects of dementia care. People who convince themselves they're lousy with finances often wind up making bad decisions. Rather, stay organized and focused so that you can eventually devote your resources to your loved one's quality of life.

Lesson 4: Minimize Chances for Sibling Disputes

Strategies

1. Hold a family conference soon after a dementia diagnosis or clear signs of impairment, addressing issues about when and how future decisions will be made, how each sibling will contribute to the situation, how financial and legal issues will be handled, and what safety considerations need to be made.
2. Encourage everyone to educate themselves about dementia, be involved to the extent they're able and desire, and respect differences of opinion.

4

THE NURSING HOME:
UNREALISTIC EXPECTATIONS

We, as a society, seem to have developed a team sport mentality of criticizing and stigmatizing our country's nursing homes, so you might be surprised to learn how far they have come in a relatively short period of time. Before the nineteenth century, no age-restricted institutions existed for long-term care. Elderly people who needed shelter because of impoverishment, incapacity, or family isolation usually ended up in an almshouse, where they lived with the homeless, the drunks, and the "insane." In 1880, one-third of the national almshouse population was made up of elderly people, a proportion that rose to 67 percent by 1923.

A symbol of failure and despair, the almshouse in 1929 was said to "stand as a threatening symbol of the deepest humiliation and degradation before all wage earners after the prime of life."[1] While legislation in 1954 allowed for the development of public institutions for the most needy older adults, it wasn't until passage of Medicare and Medicaid legislation in 1965 that the nursing home industry grew dramatically.[2] As the percentage of the population over 85 has continued to grow, nursing home care has become an increasingly common reality for many older adults. In fact, today a 65-year-old woman has almost a 50 percent chance of requiring nursing home care at some point in the future, compared with a little over 25 percent for a 65-year-old man.

Several recent trends related to our country's nursing homes are worth exploring. First of all, they are becoming much more culturally and ethnically diverse. A 2011 Brown University study found that from 1999 to 2008, there was a 6.1 percent decline in our country's total nursing home population, to 1.2 million people. However, while the number of whites in our nursing homes decreased in that time period by 10.2 percent, the number of African Americans increased by 10.8 percent. Even more strikingly, the number of

Hispanics increased by 54.9 percent, similar to the 54.1 percent rise in the Asian nursing home population.[3]

I believe this shifting of the ethnic mix in nursing homes in part reflects rates of dementia. For example, according to the 2011 Alzheimer's Disease Facts and Figures report by the Alzheimer's Association, older African Americans are probably about twice as likely to have Alzheimer's disease (AD) and other dementias as older whites, and Hispanics are about 1.5 times as likely. No known genetic factors can account for these differences across racial groups, but higher rates of diabetes and high blood pressure undoubtedly play a role.[4]

Another trend is the cultural transformation of many nursing homes in which the resident is the center of care, the environment is more homelike, and front-line staff are acknowledged and praised for their daily work with residents. My observations lead me to conclude that for many nursing homes, this transformation is still in its infancy.

Today's nursing home residents are sicker and suffering from more complex problems than ever before. In 2004, the percentage of residents with multiple physical illnesses had grown to 67 percent, while nearly 40 percent suffered from both physical and mental conditions, up from only 25 percent in 1999.[5] Consider the following resident, and then we will explore the complexities involved.

CASE STUDY

H. S. is an 82-year-old married white man with a nine-year history of Parkinson's disease. In addition to Parkinson's, he has a history of dementia, high cholesterol, degenerative joint disease, colon cancer, and bladder stones. The Parkinson's disease developed prior to the onset of dementia, and the motor symptoms related to his Parkinson's disease are under good control with medications and regular follow-up visits with a local neurologist. His dementia is considered moderate in severity (he scores 17/30 on the Mini-Mental Status Examination [MMSE], a widely used screening instrument for dementia), but his behavioral problems are significant: he engages in frequent public masturbation; urinates on stairwells, cabinets and rugs; and leers at female residents. He is a retired engineer, happily married with no children, and has no unusual sexual history. Other than a brief course of psychoanalysis 50 years ago, he has never seen a mental health professional. On exam, he displays severe memory deficits and inattention, and he minimizes and underestimates his sexual behaviors but acknowledges fantasies and a high libido.

Attempts are made to encourage the staff to intervene without resorting to medications: redirection and distraction, encouraging activity participation, and modified clothing. Despite these interventions, a decision is made in consultation with the patient's wife and primary care physician to begin treatment with oral estrogen. In several studies and case reports, use of this female hormone in men with dementia-related hypersexual behaviors has been shown to be helpful but is usually considered a last resort. Results for H. S. are good, with substantial improvement in symptoms described earlier.

In H. S. as well as other nursing home residents, the following factors influence mood and behavior:

Biologic factors: chronic illnesses, acute illnesses, sensory deficits, metabolic and
  nutritional factors, medications, and drug-drug interactions
Environmental factors: recent losses (grief), lack of privacy, strength of support
  system, financial stressors, and prospects for rehabilitation and returning home
Constitutional factors: underlying character; lifelong personality traits, habits
  and routines; likes and dislikes; coping skills; and ability to handle adversity
Dementia-related factors: short- and long-term memory impairment, attention
  span, impaired insight and judgment, language abilities, orientation, and per-
  ceptual abilities

WHAT WE EXPECT OF NURSING HOME STAFF

Imagine what we are asking of the staff, most of whom are well-intentioned, dedicated health care professionals but often lacking in education, training, and problem-solving ability. Certified nursing aides provide most of the care for residents in nursing homes, yet they are expected to perform not just competently, but heroically: to think on their feet, manage the unpredictable, be flexible, learn from and share ideas with peers and colleagues, and provide "person-centered" care rather than "task-focused" care. Imagine the psychological and emotional pressures that accompany simple day-to-day tasks; imagine wondering every day "What if he punches me, what if I get reprimanded or 'written up' for not finishing my assignment of completing the personal care of my seven residents by lunch?" Returning to the case of H. S. described earlier, consider the impact of other sexually provocative behaviors common in nursing homes: touching the caregiver in a sexually suggestive manner, propositioning staff, requesting unnecessary genital care.

DEMENTIA IN THE NURSING HOME

Developing Alzheimer's disease is a primary reason that a person gets admitted to a nursing home. Forty-two of the top 50 nursing home chains have residential Alzheimer's or memory care units, and as of December 2009 there were 83,796 special care nursing home beds dedicated to Alzheimer's disease.

At a small medical meeting in Germany in 1906, Dr. Alois Alzheimer presented the challenging case of Auguste D., a 51-year-old woman who suffered from a rapidly failing memory, confusion, disorientation, and difficulty expressing her thoughts. These symptoms did not fit any known diagnosis at the time, and in fact Auguste died after four years of steady decline that left her bedridden and mute. An autopsy showed that her brain had dramatic atrophy (shrinkage), widespread dead and dying cells, and two kinds of microscopic deposits that became known as "plaques" and "tangles." In Dr. Alzheimer's original case report from 1907, it was Auguste's psychiatric symptoms that were emphasized: "The first noticeable symptom of illness was suspiciousness of her husband . . . believing that people were out to murder her." She "screams that her husband wants to cut her open; at times, she seems to have auditory hallucinations."[6]

How incredible that more than 100 years later, we still have an illness that is often so startling and unpredictable in its manifestations. In a January 2009 review article in *Annals of Long-Term Care*, the authors noted that nursing assistants working in long-term care facilities have the highest incidence of workplace violence of any American worker, with 27 percent of all workplace violence occurring in nursing homes. Repetitive patterns of aggressive disruptive behavior were noted to occur regularly in 43 to 85 percent of nursing homes surveyed, and staff surveillance studies show that 70 percent of nursing home staff are assaulted at least monthly. Certified nursing assistants (CNAs) are physically assaulted nine times per month on average. These behaviors so well known to nursing home staff include biting, grabbing, hitting, kicking, punching and scratching. Verbally agitated and aggressive behaviors are even more common, including insults, racial slurs, swearing, accusing, and sexual advances.[7]

What is often surprising to me is the extent to which CNAs take the abuse, in effect chalking it up to their chosen career and the illnesses they are dealing with. They will laugh it off, or just appreciate the opportunity to tell someone like me about what really happens during their attempts to bathe someone, as opposed to the jargon "resistance to care" that gets transmitted in the medical chart. Studies have estimated that as many as 80 percent of incidents of aggression by patients are not reported. Other reasons proposed for such underreporting include peer pressure, cumbersome reporting policies, and fear of accusations of inadequate job performance. My feeling is that acceptance of assault as part of the job is the number one reason for such high levels of underreporting; it is a badge of honor worn by these underpaid and overworked health care professionals.

STAFF EDUCATION AND DEMENTIA–RELATED BEHAVIORS

While it is true that education and training are often helpful in curbing agitation and aggression, they are by no means a panacea. One study found that behavioral management skills training of CNAs reduced assaults by about 45 percent in the immediate posttraining period.[8] Other studies show that only 45 to 65 percent of CNAs have received training on how to handle agitated residents, and effects wear off with time unless training continues. Finally, staff education and training are often futile in view of the high turnover rates in nursing homes: annual staff turnover rates range from 25 to 150 percent. This means that if a staff of 40 people has an annual turnover rate of 50 percent, only 20 of those 40 staff members will still be working at the facility in a year. Staff turnover is, of course, largely influenced by staff satisfaction, which in turn is largely influenced by workload. An interesting study published in the *Gerontologist* in 2006 collected data from 854 nursing homes in six states to examine the association between staff turnover and organizational characteristics. For-profit ownership, lower staffing levels, and lower quality of care were associated with higher turnover, while smaller nursing home size was associated with lower turnover.[9] I have personally found this to be valid: the homes that I visit regularly and in which I see the same CNAs and nurses for years tend to be the smaller, family-owned or religiously affiliated homes with close community ties that generally have more staff with solid job satisfaction. Amazingly, a 2001 study conducted by the Centers for Medicare and Medicaid (CMS) found that for nurses aides, staffing levels in more than 91 percent of skilled nursing facilities (SNFs) were below levels deemed minimally necessary to provide care in dressing and grooming, exercise, feeding assistance, changing wet clothes, positioning, and providing toileting.

In addition to agitation and aggression directed at nursing home staff, there is another category of behavior problems that is less publicized and less well understood: violence *between* residents. Mark S. Lachs, MD, referring to aggression between residents during a recent symposium on the subject held at the annual meeting of the Gerontological Society of America, "The most prevalent form of elder mistreatment in long-term care has been virtually unexplored and unstudied."[10] In one focus group study involving seven residents and 96 staff members of a large, urban nursing home, virtually all staff members reported seeing or experiencing resident-resident aggression (RRA). These incidents were most frequent in dining rooms and residents' rooms, and in the afternoon, although they occurred regularly throughout the facility at all times. Interventions included changing a resident's room, physically intervening and separating residents, and removing a resident from the dining room or other public area and changing seating arrangements there. Triggers of these incidents included disputes over control of the television or possession of a newspaper, rummaging through or taking other residents' belongings, and wandering into other residents' rooms. In my experience, dining room incidents are so common that I once put together a 45-minute lecture on the topic for the inpatient geriatric psychiatry unit staff at Butler Hospital, Brown University's primary psychiatric training facility. Tensions mount in the dining areas: residents bicker, they get upset when a tablemate engages in socially inappropriate behaviors (e.g., grunting, picking noses, pouring drinks on the table), and they get overwhelmed by the noise, the trays with too many individually wrapped items to cope with, and waiting for the food. One resident taking another's food may trigger an outburst.

A fascinating research project called CareMedia, based at Carnegie Mellon University's School of Computer Science and funded by the National Science

Foundation, is developing automated video and sensor analysis tools to "provide better insight into the lives of nursing home residents."[11] In a pilot study involving nine residents of one nursing home's dementia unit, the researchers collected 320 camera hours of data from four video cameras and then analyzed 188 of those hours. The results were startling. The cameras recorded dozens of acts of physical aggression by residents, including slapping, kicking, grabbing, punching, and scratching. In 30 of the recorded incidents, the target was another resident, in 20 it was a staff member, and in 15 the aggression was directed at an object. In 40 percent of the events, there was an observable event to which the perpetrator was responding, and nearly half the incidents had not been witnessed by staff.

These preliminary results, while extremely important in verifying the extent of the problem, do not shock me. Compounding the situation is of course the lack of staff education about dementia. Instead of the behavior being rightfully attributed to the dementia, residents may be judged, labeled, or categorized as "defiant, manipulative, nasty, impossible." To cope with the stress, fear, and uncertainty elicited by these residents, staff may knowingly or unknowingly act out by ignoring needs, making degrading comments or joking at the residents' expense, or arguing with residents despite its futility.

One aspect of nursing homes that I've always marveled at is the degree with which nurses and aides working with the *same residents* differ so dramatically in their characterizations of those residents. How is it possible that a resident is described as "mean, defiant, attention-seeking, aware of everything that goes on" by one CNA who works with that resident on a daily basis, while another CNA on a different shift says, "We get along great. I never have a problem with her," and "She's pretty confused"? I have several possible explanations for these discrepancies. First of all, we tend to underestimate the degree to which residents with dementia fluctuate in their symptoms from day to day. Fluctuations in lucidity, for example, are often mystifying to the staff, who conclude that the only rational explanation for this is that the resident is somehow "doing this on purpose to get attention." In fact, the dementia-related increase in behavioral symptoms that occurs in the early evening hours (sundowning) is a real phenomenon. Probable explanations include fatigue, decrease in structured activities as the day progresses, and overstimulation and chaos associated with shift change. I've been present in nursing home dementia units in which the same resident who was calm, pleasant, engaging, and affable at 11 A.M. was angry, restless, labile and unredirectable at 4 P.M.

Second, we fail to appreciate the often chaotic lives and personal problems that CNAs bring with them to the workplace. In his 1998 book *Senior Living Communities: Operations Management and Marketing for Assisted Living, Congregate, and Continuing Care Retirement Communities* (JHU Press), Benjamin W. Pearce, president and chief executive officer of Potomac Homes Corporation, writes: "At the very bottom of the totem pole is the certified nursing assistant (CNA). It has always been a mystery to me where that name came from; if anything, the nurses are assisting the CNAs, who really do all the work. Many of them are poorly educated and unskilled, and they have their share of personal problems. The CNA job is without a doubt one of the toughest there is, tantamount to indoor manual labor. It is emotionally and physically draining, and the pay is usually poor."[12] Mr. Pearce is right on the mark, and I vividly recall a well-regarded CNA approaching me in the stairwell of the nursing home to plead for advice regarding her abusive husband. Many others, including nurses, aides, dining staff, and housekeeping staff have asked me to help with their family conflicts, depression, and even managing their psychiatric medications. Imagine the immense challenge faced by someone whose own personal relationships are often embroiled in arguments and insults to then transition to the workplace, where those same patterns are now being inflicted on them by people whose personal care they are now responsible for. Yet many of these dedicated and hardworking professionals are doing the best they can under adverse circumstances. Consider this quote from Pearce's book: "CNAs can not simply be motivated by the pay they earn. If they are given the right amount of supportive management and recognition, they will stay. Over time a symbiotic relationship will develop between patients and their CNAs. Patients will tell the CNAs how much they appreciate them, comment on their appearance, help them through their personal problems, and even love them. Each becomes a support system for the other, and it is then in the CNAs' best interests to care for their patients." I've seen residents develop episodes of grief-related clinical depression when their longstanding CNA leaves the facility for another job or for some other reason.

Unfortunately, violence in the nursing home is here to stay. Although federal guidelines require reporting to nursing home administrators and state health departments all incidents of mistreatment, neglect, abuse, and misappropriation of resident property, incidents of resident-resident aggression create special challenges. As noted by Jeanne A. Teresi, EdD, PhD, of Columbia University in a recent interview: "When there are two residents involved, it's a little more vague. When at least one is cognitively impaired, who are the perpetrator and the victim?"[13]

What surprises me is that there aren't more episodes of serious violence between residents in nursing homes. In 2002, more than 3,700 complaints about such aggression were lodged with state ombudsman programs, up from about 2,500 in 1997. In 2008, I was asked to be an expert witness in a case of resident-resident aggression in a nursing home that resulted in the death of the victim. Both residents, who were roommates, had dementia. In the weeks leading up to the final act of severe violence, there were three separate documented verbal arguments between the two residents. In one, they "yelled at each other" because one was rummaging through the other's closet and putting on his clothes. Paranoia was a factor, a symptom discussed in more depth in Chapter 1. Certainly interventions designed to prevent, anticipate, and better deal with such violence and lessen its impact will be a welcome outcome of studies such as the CareMedia research cited previously.

CONSISTENT ASSIGNMENT

One concept in nursing home staffing that I believe is especially helpful for residents with dementia is consistent assignment. Consistent assignment means that residents see the same caregivers (registered nurse, licensed practical nurse, or certified nursing assistant) almost every time these professionals are on duty. Most residents are more comfortable and calmer with caregivers who know them well and understand their personality quirks, personal preferences, and unique needs. This type of staffing model not only benefits the residents but also leads to reduced staff turnover and increased staff satisfaction. Staff who take care of the same residents are happier in their jobs and tend to stay in their jobs. Reasons for resistance to this type of staffing include management's desire for fairness, so they rotate staff so that they become familiar with the needs of all the residents in the building or unit, as well as a desire to prevent staff burnout.

THE NURSING HOME SOCIAL WORKER

In my view, there is nothing that illustrates our dysfunctional system of dementia care in nursing homes more than the nursing home social worker. As person-centered dementia care has become accepted as the gold standard, who else is better equipped to set the framework for that individualized care? When I am asked to evaluate a nursing home resident, regardless of the reason (depression, anxiety, agitation, etc.), I turn first to the social work section of the chart. It is here that the scene is set for my visit: the resident's life story should be presented so that the reader appreciates the *person* who is behind the cognitively impaired *patient*. His or her place of birth, number of siblings, level of schooling, marital status, number of children, and occupational history are presented, along with his or her hobbies, favorite television shows, places travelled, personality quirks, and so on. The better social workers will also comment on the quality of the resident's relationships, his or her social support network, strategies of coping with stress, and so on. The National Association of Social Workers (NASW), the country's largest social work membership organization, states that a nursing home social services director should be a graduate of a master's degree program from an accredited school or program of social work and have a minimum of two years postgraduate experience in long-term care or related settings. In reality, this seems to be the exception rather than the rule. A 2004 study of 87 long-term care facilities in the Midwest reported that only 36 percent of nursing homes employed a social worker who would be considered qualified by NASW standards.[14]

Another 2004 study found that 11 percent of nursing homes with more than 120 beds did not employ a qualified social worker and were out of federal compliance.[15] Inexplicably, the federal government doesn't require nursing home social workers to have a social work degree, unlike federal regulations in other settings such as hospice, the Veterans Administration (VA) nursing home system, and home health. In the nursing home setting, the federal government considers a "qualified social worker" a person with a bachelor's degree in social work or another human service field with one year supervised experience in a health-related setting. State laws are even more lax: the Administrative Code in many states does not require nursing homes with fewer than 121 beds to even employ a social worker. In a study published in 2009, data were collected from a national sample of 1,071 nursing home social service directors in 2006. The results were startling: among them, only 38 percent of social service directors were licensed in social work, and more than two-thirds of the respondents did not belong to a professional organization that would help them stay connected to their field.[16] Yet consider what realistic expectations are for a nursing home social worker: to facilitate communication between staff, residents, and families; to comprehensively assess residents and match them with the facilities' resources to maximize their independence and quality of life; and to involve the local community in the facility. I also count on social workers to be liaisons when problems arise that need to involve the state ombudsman for long-term care or when questions of a resident's mental capacity arise that may involve a separate assessment of mental capacity to be used in legal guardianship proceedings. Finally, I assume that the nursing home professional most prepared to foster a healthy psychosocial environment and to screen residents for depression, anxiety, and memory deficits is the social worker.

Over the years, I have dutifully and faithfully preached what I (and others) know to be the best strategies for managing agitation and aggression in dementia, those that don't involve medications (Table 4.1). These types of recommendations are sensible, practical, and cost-effective. Yet without qualified staff in place,

Table 4.1
Practical Suggestions for Decreasing Agitation and Aggression in Dementia

Communicate Effectively	Decrease Escalation	Review the Basics
• Capture the person's attention: stay in view • Use simple, direct statements • Limit choices • Use gestures to assist with verbal instructions • Speak clearly and slowly; allow time for response • Lower tone if voice needs to be raised • Make known your desire to help	• Approach in a calm manner • Use distraction: food, drink, music, conversation • Maintain eye contact and comfortable posture • Match verbal and nonverbal signals • Identify and state the affect observed in the patient • Identify what is triggering the behavior • Modify the environment	• Separate the behavior from the person • Know the person and structure the environment accordingly • Don't minimize the importance of a loving voice, attentiveness, touch, and consistency • Maintain the patient's religious and spiritual identity

how realistic are they to implement in the heat of the moment, when tensions are high and the situations require split-second thinking and effective problem-solving skills that would challenge even the most accomplished clinician?

MEDICATIONS FOR AGITATION AND AGGRESSION

I can confidently say that nursing homes aren't exactly among the most admired and revered institutions in our country. Now imagine the pressures that nursing homes are under to minimize medication use for dementia-related behavioral problems. The *Wall Street Journal* ran a page one story on December 4, 2007, entitled "Prescription Abuse Seen in U.S. Nursing Homes." Statistics from CMS were cited that showed nearly 30 percent of the total nursing home population is receiving antipsychotic drugs, yet most of these residents suffered from dementia as opposed to the true psychotic illnesses that these drugs are indicated by the U.S. Food and Drug Administration (FDA) for. Experts acknowledge that there are few effective medicines to manage the outbursts of Alzheimer's patients. To make matters worse, in April 2005 the FDA issued an advisory and subsequent black box warning that elderly patients with dementia-related psychosis treated with the newer (atypical) antipsychotic drugs are at an increased risk (1.6 to 1.7 times) of death compared with placebo (4.5% versus 2.6% respectively).

The easy answer is to continue to vilify the pharmaceutical industry as greedy evil-doers and reserve antipsychotics as strictly treatments of last resort or for humanitarian purposes. Even geriatrician Joshua D. Schor, MD, in his 2008 book *The Nursing Home Guide* wrote that in the specialized dementia units of the nursing home where he practices, "We use fewer medications even if it means more residents with aggressive behaviors."[17] He apparently believes that in most cases the risks of these medications outweigh the potential benefits. But this belief ignores scientific data: a 2006 Cochrane review on the use of atypical antipsychotics for agitation and psychosis in individuals with Alzheimer's disease found that risperidone (Risperdal) significantly improved both conditions, while olanzapine (Zyprexa) improved only agitation.[18] There are also risks of *not* providing medications for nursing home residents with dementia-related behavioral problems: falling, being ostracized by the staff and other residents, suffering adverse health impacts from refusing care and medications, among others. The American Psychiatric Association's revised practice guideline for the treatment of patients with Alzheimer's and other dementias notes that "Appropriate use of antipsychotic medications can relieve symptoms and reduce distress and can increase safety for patients, other residents, and staff."[19]

What recourse does the nursing home have when behaviors escalate to the point that the staff "can't take it anymore"? You guessed it: the inpatient geriatric psychiatry unit. The decision to "send someone out" is often subjective and influenced by a host of factors unrelated to the true clinical need. These factors include the resident's medical insurance, the current bed availability of the hospital, the stress level (i.e., need for a brief respite) of the staff, and the threshold of the facility for tolerating difficult behaviors. Some facilities are fortunate enough to "pick and choose" their residents to ensure minimal presence of problem behaviors, while others "take whatever they can get," including severely behaviorally impaired residents, those with personality and substance use disorders, and those with chronic psychiatric illnesses that previously had been cared for in group homes and state psychiatric facilities. Unfortunately, as lengths of stays have declined and medical and psychosocial complexities have increased, the inpatient unit is all too often an unsatisfying experience for all concerned (see Chapter 7 for details).

The January 2007 issue of the *AARP Magazine* offers 10 essential tips for selecting a nursing home for a loved one, including "getting the list (of nursing homes in your area)," "popping in unannounced," "looking close to home," and "checking out the food and drink."[20] Interestingly, none of the 10 AARP tips mention dementia. Even nursing homes themselves are often in denial about the extent to which their residents have dementia. Consider the American Health Care Association's consumer guide "Living In a Nursing Home: Myths and Realities."[21] The second myth is: that nursing facility patients are confused. I would argue that that is a reality more than a myth.

Another important and underrecognized factor that greatly affects nursing home staff is interacting with difficult families. Not surprisingly, having to send a loved one to a nursing home seems to bring out the worst in people. The guilt, the stress of the resident's illness, the unplanned, often crisislike circumstances of the admission, and the faulty health care system that provides so little support or education to families all converge to maximize distress. Never mind the data that firmly establish the immense caregiver burden in dementia, such as the 75 percent of caregivers that report feeling depressed and the 66 percent that have significant depression. It is after admission that dysfunctional patterns of family behaviors often emerge, draining the staff of energy and taking precious time away from resident care. Patterns may include overinvolvement (dictating which medications to use or refusing medications altogether), splitting (playing one staff member against another), instigation, harassment, intimidation, and indecision or unavailability. For example, while family members are encouraged to participate in care plan meetings with the staff, one of the statements I come across most frequently in residents' charts is "Family was invited to the care plan meeting but chose not to attend." One nursing home I visited was so overwhelmed by difficult families that they convinced me to put together an inservice program to offer suggestions. My suggestions included the following:

1. Identify the primary decision maker.
2. Designate a family spokesperson.
3. Invite and encourage family to attend care conference.
4. Set mutual expectations and rules.
5. Incorporate family maladjustment into care plan.

6. Provide emotional support.
7. Consider referral for family assessment and interventions.

Before moving on to exploring assisted living facilities, let's review the primary "reality lessons" learned about dementia in nursing home residents and how to translate those lessons into practical, realistic strategies to maximize both the caregiver and the resident's quality of life.

LESSON 1: COMPLEXITY OF RESIDENTS WITH DEMENTIA

Strategies

1. Help gather medical and psychiatric *records* from doctors, hospitals, and other institutions.
2. If off-site *consultants* are needed and requested (e.g., neurology, neuropsychology, or internal medicine subspecialties), ensure that records and a clear reason for referral are sent. A family member or staff member who knows the resident should accompany him or her to the appointment if at all possible.
3. Explore the extent of *behavioral health/psychiatric services* in the facility, including visit frequency, availability of psychotherapy services, and family communication. This is not just my personal bias as a geriatric psychiatrist. Consider the following, taken from the May 2009 article "Quality of Medical Care in British Care Homes." "Support for patients with dementia also seems to be lacking. Up to 75 percent of residents in care homes have dementia. The National Dementia strategy suggests a specialist mental health assessment on admission and regular review . . ."[22]

LESSON 2: POORLY EDUCATED STAFF

Strategies

1. Ask administrator and directors of nursing and social services what educational programs are offered to staff.
2. Make it known that dementia training and education are important to you and your family. Suggestions may include inservice programs, lectures by local dementia experts or Alzheimer's Association staff, or group viewing of the HBO Alzheimer's documentary series.

LESSON 3: HIGH STAFF TURNOVER

Strategy

Ask an administrator or director of nursing to comment on staff turnover and steps taken to minimize it.

Lesson 4: High Levels of Aggressive/Violent Behaviors

Strategies

1. Accept its inevitability to some degree.
2. Ensure steps are taken by staff to minimize incidents: nonpharmacologic strategies, medications when appropriate, anticipating problems and intervening early, and so on.
3. Be honest and open at admission about triggers of agitation or aggression in your loved one, including the presence of paranoia, anger outbursts at home, and so on. Worry less about hurt feelings and more about the safety of residents and staff.

Lesson 5: Day-to-Day Fluctuations and Sundowning

Sundowning refers to a variety of difficult behaviors in dementia that tend to occur at a regular time each day, usually in the early evening. The behaviors may include increased confusion, disorientation, hallucinations, agitation, and aggression. Possible explanations include afternoon fatigue, caregiver fatigue, and too much stimulation in the environment. In a nursing home, for example, sundowning often occurs around 3 P.M., when shifts change and there is more noise and general chaos.

Strategies

1. Summarize (in writing) regular, predictable patterns of confusion, agitation, and/or restlessness that occurred prior to the nursing home admission. Present this summary at a care plan meeting.
2. Provide tips for staff in managing symptoms (e.g., stuffed animals, soft music, using iPods, leafing through photos or cards, playing video tapes of loved ones, or providing reassurance and comforting messages). Sometimes providing natural sun exposure in the morning or using bright light therapy may be helpful.

Lesson 6: Importance of Social Worker

Strategies

1. Meet and have a conversation about the social worker's background, style, and educational degree. Acknowledge his or her role as highly important and valued member of the treatment team.
2. Prepare background information about your loved one for the social worker so that it can be easily incorporated into his or her assessment.

LESSON 7: KEEPING EXPECTATIONS REALISTIC

Strategies

1. Acknowledge that while you expect high quality care, you are *realistic* and don't expect miracles. Acting in a litigious and reprimanding manner usually decreases the chances of high-quality care.
2. Be respectful and understanding of the challenging and stressful work performed in nursing homes.

LESSON 8: HELPING WITH BATHING

Helping your loved one with Alzheimer's disease with bathing is arguably the most challenging aspect of caregiving that the nursing home staff will face. You should feel empowered to do what you can to help the staff with this difficult task. The following strategies are meant to minimize distress and the need for medications during the bathing process.

Strategies

1. Consider dignity and modesty first and foremost. Issues of privacy, modesty, and humility play major roles in the bathing process. It may help for your loved one to start the bath with some of his or her clothes on (such as a t-shirt or undershirt). A caregiver with a steady, confident, and reassuring approach may also help.
2. Realize there are options: tub bath, bed bath, or shower. Tub baths are good for skin care needs, while showers have the advantage of a hand-held shower nozzle to avoid spray hitting the face. Bed baths are done more often in later-stage dementia, when anxiety, agitation, and aggression are more severe and easily precipitated by a shower or tub bath.
3. Keep the bathing experience as calm and unhurried as possible. Having your loved one hold an item such as soap or shampoo may help him or her feel safe and connected to the bathing process. Be willing to change approaches, since what worked yesterday may not work today.

LESSON 9: USING MEDICARE'S FIVE-STAR QUALITY RATING SYSTEM

The Five-Star Quality Rating System (available at www.medicare.gov/NHCompare) was created to help caregivers compare nursing homes more easily. With detailed information about every Medicare- and Medicaid-certified nursing home in the country, separate ratings are provided for three areas: health inspections, staffing, and quality measures. For example, a home may get three out of five stars for health inspections, four out of five stars for staffing, and two out of five stars for quality measures. There is also an overall rating, which combines the three ratings.

Strategies

1. Don't rely too much on these ratings. For example, don't use this tool to try to compare a nursing home in one state with one in another state. In addition, the staffing data are self-reported by the nursing home and are reported just once a year. The quality measures, while interesting to look at, represent only a few of the many aspects of care that may be important in your situation.
2. Rather than getting caught up in the number of stars a home receives, look for red flags instead. For example, one home I looked at on the website received several administrative deficiencies, including failing to choose a doctor to be the medical director and failing to even hire a properly licensed administrator.
3. Keep in mind that nowhere in the ratings is there specific information about management of dementia. But focus on the items that are most relevant to you and your situation. For example, if your loved one already has a poor appetite, when he or she is ready to move into a nursing home, it will be important to look at the percentage of long-stay residents who lose too much weight.

5

THE ASSISTED LIVING FACILITY: PRISTINE LIVING WITH A CATCH

The words "nursing home" are met with a negative response from most people, often those with little or no personal experience with these facilities. The images conjured are typically bleak: stark, desolate institutions where residents are warehoused with little hope for a reasonable quality of life. Experts and elder care websites alike urge people to never promise a loved one you won't put them in a nursing home because it's a promise you may not be able to keep. Many baby boomers recall the nursing home scandals of the late 1970s, when harsh chemical and physical restraints were often the norm, and the federal government was compelled to act by instituting the Omnibus Budget Reconciliation Act (OBRA) Guidelines in 1987. These guidelines—including regulations for behavioral, environmental, medication, and restraint standards—were the first of many regulations that have led to the nursing home industry being one of the most heavily regulated industries in the United States. I find it ironic that the country's recent financial collapse has in part been attributed to lax regulations of recent years, yet clearly the nursing home industry is an example of how overregulation doesn't necessarily fix the underlying problems.

In contrast, the assisted living industry has largely escaped such stigma and negative public perception. Experts never recommend against saying, "I promise I'll never put you in a really nice assisted living facility with a bar and a fitness center."

HISTORY AND REGULATION OF ASSISTED LIVING FACILITIES

Assisted living emerged in the late 1980s and early 1990s as the next step of continuing care for people who can no longer live independently in their own home but who do not require the 24-hour medical care provided by a nursing home. Negative views of nursing homes and changing values regarding living environments for seniors contributed to the assisted living movement, and Wall Street money fueled their expansion in the mid 1990s.

There is no nationally recognized definition of assisted living. Assisted living facilities (ALFs) are regulated and licensed at the state level. More than two-thirds of states use the licensure term "assisted living." Other terms intended to relay this same level of care include "residential care home," "assisted care living facilities," and "personal care homes." Each state licensing agency has its own definition of the term it uses to describe assisted living. Assisted living can refer to services that are licensed as residential care facilities, homes for the aged, and personal care homes, with the basic element being some combination of housing and personal care. Unlike nursing homes and other institutionalized long-term care settings, assisted living is unique in its emphasis on a philosophy of providing residents with varying levels of choice and independence. Ideally, an assisted living facility provides a homelike environment that minimizes the need to move when the services a resident requires increase. Not only is independence fostered, so are autonomy, dignity, and privacy.

According to one study, there were 36,451 licensed assisted living facilities with 937,601 beds in 2004. Although ALF growth was flat through 2004, demand was as strong or stronger in 2006 than in 2005. Based on 2008 data and ranked by total assisted living occupant capacity, the top three companies were Sunrise Senior Living, Emeritus Corp., and Brookdale Senior Living. Despite the credit crisis and financial meltdown that have taken a heavy toll on the real estate industry, assisted living services continue to expand. Hospice care has also become more popular, with 24 companies offering the service to residents in 2008, compared with 16 in 2007.[1]

Hospice care may be beneficial to assisted living residents with dementia and their caregivers, but it is still a relatively new phenomenon. For example, pet therapy and music therapy, in addition to the reassuring, friendly voices that accompany hospice care, may be used effectively by hospice workers who are helping residents with dementia. One 2009 study found that the quality and nature of resident-staff and assisted living-hospice staff relationships were critical in promoting good end-of-life care for ALF residents on hospice.[2] Many hospice programs offer grief and bereavement counseling for families as well.

The growing popularity of assisted living has led to design innovations that have arguably benefited many residents with dementia. For example, it was on an ALF dementia unit that I first saw, instead of the words "rest room" on the bathroom door, a picture of a toilet instead. Other areas of design innovation include lighting, porches, looped walking pathways, social living spaces, and gardens and outdoor environments.

Unlike nursing homes, ALFs are regulated by the states, not the federal government. Although the assisted living industry is much less heavily regulated than the nursing home industry, efforts are afoot to change that. More than one-third of states updated their assisted living regulations in 2008, while

10 indicated that major changes to regulations were underway or slated for 2009, according to the *2009 Assisted Living State Regulatory Review*, published annually by the National Centers for Assisted Living. At least 18 states reported making statutory, regulatory, or policy changes in 2010 and January 2011. Specific trends that occurred in 2008 included five states that increased or modified medication management standards, and four states that added or changed background check requirements.[3]

Evaluating the quality of assisted living facilities is easier said than done. Consider the following statement from a 2007 article published in the *Gerontologist*: "Any meaningful concept of 'quality' must embrace a variety of dimensions, including quality of care, quality of life, the physical environment, and resident rights. The ability to use a multidimensional concept of quality is complicated by the lack of consensus, confusion, and disagreement among consumers, providers, and regulators about the role of assisted living. This disagreement significantly confounds the task of comparing quality among assisted living settings and between assisted living and other types of long-term care."[4]

COST AND PAYMENT ISSUES IN ASSISTED LIVING

Cost and payment source are another major difference between assisted living facilities and nursing homes. As a residential service with 24-hour care, nursing homes remain the most costly option for long-term institutional care, with fees now approaching and sometimes even exceeding $100,000 per year. Most of those costs are covered by Medicaid, which contributes to fiscal crises in many states. In contrast, the majority of assisted living residents pay from their own financial resources, although 41 states offer waiver programs that allow low-income residents to reside in assisted living.

Medication management in particular deserves mention here, largely because the need for assistance with complex medication regimens is often one factor that leads to ALF admission. I've seen many patients who, despite being capable of managing most of their affairs independently, had no idea what medications they were taking or what they were for. So you would think that of all the health-related services provided by assisted living facilities, medication management would be perfected. But in reality it's often inadequate. Important issues that turn up include medication delivery by unlicensed personnel, as well as the lack of systems in place to monitor medication safety. In some states, the laws are vague regarding which staff members may assist with medication management in an ALF, and nearly half the states permit registered nurses (RNs) to delegate the administration of oral medications, if not other drugs, to aides. In fact, a multistate survey of licensing officials regarding sources of ALF deficiencies and complaints found that the leading sources of concern were medication administration issues and staffing issues. In keeping with a theme in this chapter that in many ways the residents of assisted living facilities are just as complex as the residents of nursing homes, it's interesting to note that the number of medications taken by ALF residents actually rivals the number taken by skilled nursing facility residents. Yet the undertreatment of some common medical problems in ALF residents points to the emphasis on the social model of assisted living as opposed to the medical model. For example, a recent study in four states involving over 2,000 residents found that in 172 residents with a prior heart attack, 60 percent were not receiving aspirin, and 76 percent were not receiving beta blockers. Studies have shown that for people who have had a prior heart attack, the use of aspirin, beta blockers, and lipid-lowering drugs reduces the risk of recurrent heart attack and death. Similarly, more than half of the residents with osteoporosis were not receiving any treatment for it.[5]

For many facilities, balancing the social and medical aspects of life for their elderly residents is a tricky business. I remember one facility with an elegant restaurantlike dining area whose menu and sophisticated decor could easily have earned it a respectable Zagat guide rating. Now imagine that while most of the residents were enjoying their lunch and waiting for the dessert course to arrive, a woman who had finished her lunch an hour earlier at the previous seating reappeared at her table, demanding to be seated for the lunch that she couldn't recall having just finished. While such behavior in a nursing home would likely be hardly noticed, in assisted living it can have far-reaching implications.

Residents often form cliques, talking with other clique members in hushed tones about "that lady over there who doesn't know what she's doing." They may comment about how the man they used to play bridge with is "now on the locked ward," referring to the secure dementia special care unit that the facility may have. A 2006 paper entitled "Conflicts, Friendship Cliques, and Territorial Displays in Senior Center Environments" showed how common dining area territorial conflicts were, and how territories supported group identity and interaction for friends who shared dining tables.[6]

In an article in the *Arizona Republic*, a woman describes being bullied for the first time in her life at age 76 after moving to a retirement community in Arizona. "There is a clique here that is meaner than mean," she says, as she reports being chased away from seats at the community pool. The article notes that "dementia may provoke such nasty behavior," which makes sense since bullying is usually a response to someone or something that makes people with dementia feel insecure. Robin Bonifas, who is researching bullying at the University of Arizona, estimates that 10 to 20 percent of older people in care homes experience some type of abuse from fellow residents. She gets it right when she says that "the best way to deal with bullying is to have an all-around culture where bullying is unacceptable."[7]

Just as nursing home staff are expected to perform heroically with their medically and behaviorally complex residents on a daily basis, assisted living staff are expected to negotiate the social and interpersonal landmines that assisted living presents on a regular basis. The mere presence of a wide-screen television set in a common area can precipitate conflict, especially when residents with mild or moderate dementia are commingled with residents without cognitive impairment.

As with nursing homes, staff turnover in assisted living is troubling: the average staff turnover rate is estimated at 42 percent, with a range of 21 to 135 percent. Studies suggest that having a full-time RN on staff reduces the likelihood that ALF residents will be transferred to a nursing home. Amazingly, only 26 states require that ALFs employ or contract with nurses. Differences vary widely state to state: New Jersey, for example, requires that a nurse be available at all times (on call and reachable by phone) and directs facilities to have RNs coordinate all resident health care services. States such as Tennessee, on the other hand, require only that a nurse be available as needed. Facilities in 33 states are required to provide training on a variety of topics, although the rigor of training curriculum requirements and hours of training vary widely from state to state. With respect to dementia, at times it feels like training curriculum requirements should apply to the officials and regulators as well as the staff. In Rhode Island, for example, a recent trend has been for the state's Department of Health to identify assisted living facility residents that have cognitive deficits and dementia diagnoses and essentially *insist that they move into the secure unit of the facility.* In a recent case in which I was involved, the fact that the state official found a resident to be somewhat disoriented and confused led to a decision to transfer the resident to the secure dementia unit, despite the resident's relatively preserved functional abilities and excellent adjustment to the facility's assisted living milieu. Because of her family's opposition to the move (the secure unit residents were much more impaired and low-functioning than she was), I re-evaluated her to convince myself I was right in advocating for her to stay where she was. She expressed her contentment, telling me she "now has peace and tranquility, no stress." Despite her score of 16/30 on the Mini-Mental State Examination (MMSE) she was remarkably poised: she escorted me on a short tour of the facility, showing me the dining room and the group activity room and praising both. She never attempted to elope and never got lost attempting to find the dining room. Her activities of daily living (ADLs), including bathing, dressing and feeding required so little assistance that it really would have been absurd (not to mention detrimental to her well-being) to move her at this stage of her illness.

At least for the large segment of the industry that is private pay and caters to the more affluent, the images people have of ALFs are quite different than those of nursing homes: bright, open designs; upscale furnishings; restaurantlike dining settings. Consider the following descriptions of several continuing care retirement communities that "garner four- or five-star Medicare nursing home ratings and accreditation from the Commission on Accreditation of Rehabilitation Facilities" provided by CNNMoney.com in a February 2009 story, "Retire In Style."[8]

Westminster Village: Spanish Fort, Alabama

"Located on a 56-acre property near Mobile Bay, Westminster Village has many perks: a heated indoor pool, a woodworking shop, gardening areas, a fitness center (staffed with professional exercise physiologists), a fully equipped library and three modes of transportation."

Willamette View: Portland, Oregon

"Willamette View's most appealing amenity may be its 5,600 square foot wellness center with a pool, personal trainers, massage therapists, and a high-tech gym (residents just plug in a USB stick and the machines remember their workouts). This energetic community sustains 150 lifestyle committees and clubs including a 60-voice chorus and world affairs programs."

Nearly all ALFs surveyed in a recent study provide wellness activities, group outings, and emergency call systems to those who pay basic rates, and more than half offer nursing services and special diets to those who pay basic rates. But less than half provide medication assistance, medication administration, or help with activities of daily living (ADLs) as part of their basic package of services.[9]

In fact, many of these facilities are truly gorgeous buildings in fabulous settings: I have to chuckle when I recall the handful of assisted living residents I've seen over the years (with dementia of course) who actually believed that they were on a cruise ship or in a hotel. One gentleman would call the front desk "for room service." Nevertheless, the reality for the assisted living industry is, of course, somewhat different, with the overarching theme being "there is no escaping dementia." A January 2005 article shed light on this issue, examining 230 consenting residents in seven assisted living facilities in and around Omaha, Nebraska. None of these facilities were designated "Alzheimer's" or "dementia" facilities, yet the findings were striking. Fifty-eight percent of the residents had cognitive impairment (based on a commonly used tool for dementia screening), yet only 37 percent of these people had a diagnosis of dementia. Seventy-five percent were on no dementia treatment, 22 percent self-administered an average of 5.4 medications daily, and only 11 percent had surrogate decision makers (health care proxies).[10]

The Alzheimer's Association notes that "at least half of assisted living residents age 65 and older have Alzheimer's disease, another disease or condition that causes dementia, or cognitive impairment that is probably caused by these diseases and conditions."[11] The Maryland Assisted Living Study, conducted from 2001 to 2002, found that 68 percent of elderly assisted living residents had dementia.[12] Two-thirds had Alzheimer's disease (AD), and the remaining one-third had dementia caused by vascular and other diseases. The National Survey of Assisted Living Facilities, conducted in a national random sample of residential facilities in 1998, concluded that about one-third of elderly residents had *moderate to severe cognitive impairment* indicative of dementia. This compares with the 60 percent of nursing home residents with dementia who are in the moderate and severe stages of the illness. The study was conducted in 1,547 facilities that had 11 or more beds, primarily served elderly people, and called themselves "assisted living" or provided specified services, including 24-hour supervision.[13]

Other studies have found higher than expected rates of mood and anxiety disorders, personality disorders, and other psychiatric problems that in fact were often the *principal reason* for the residents' admission to the facility. These are not the healthy retirees that the facilities sought to attract when they were built, those elderly persons who were looking to live in beautiful settings with all the amenities.

The following case is not atypical. Several years ago I was asked to see a resident of an ALF who was living in the "independent" section of the facility. This meant the 85-year-old woman was pretty much on her own. She managed her own medications (none for dementia, of course), and she was expected to attend to her own grooming and personal hygiene as well as to negotiate the dining room schedule and the social activity schedule that was provided to her. Given her independent status, the facility staff had little to do with her, and her medical chart was virtually empty. "We don't know her" was the response of the nurse when I asked her to help me understand the resident's situation and the reason for the referral. It turned out the resident had wandered over a mile away from the building one afternoon and was brought back by the police. Fortunately, she had remained on the main road, although it was a busy thoroughfare with two-way traffic and a 45–mile per hour speed limit. When the administrator brought her son in the next day to insist she move to the "assisted living" section of the building, he resisted. "Don't worry, I'll just read her the riot act and she won't do that again, " he insisted. Needless to say, at this point he was given only two choices: move her to the assisted living section or remove her from the facility.

What is striking about this case is that it was only after a potential crisis, an act of danger, that formal assistance was sought. There was no early recognition or proactivity, no staff member who recognized that this woman was clearly disoriented and memory impaired and had no business living in the independent section of the facility. In many ways, the health care system in its dysfunctional state perpetuates the problem: if this woman had been sent to the local emergency department for evaluation, she would have undoubtedly been discharged in a couple of hours with instructions to return to the nursing home. She would have checked out fine medically: pleasantly confused, normal laboratory studies and vital signs, no infections or acute problems. And most emergency department staff have no idea what an assisted living facility really is and how it differs so dramatically from a nursing home: they would assume that she was being closely monitored by attentive nurses and aides.

The Alzheimer's Association states that "many assisted living residents with these conditions (Alzheimer's disease and other dementias) do not have a formal diagnosis, and assisted living staff members do not always recognize the conditions in their residents,"[14] and I find this to be the understatement of the year. A member of my clinical team once discovered that an elderly male assisted living resident with mild dementia and a history of depression and suicidal thoughts actually had a *machete* in his apartment.

In many respects, delivering quality behavioral health services to assisted living residents is significantly more challenging than delivering care to nursing home residents. In an enlightening 2003 study, administrators of 94 assisted living facilities in Michigan completed a 19-item survey about the extent of residents' mental health problems and how such problems were addressed. Not surprisingly, the three most commonly reported mental illnesses were dementia, depression, and hallucinations or delusions, while the three most commonly reported problematic behaviors were resistance to care, wandering, and verbal abuse. Barriers that prevented a resident from receiving mental health care were many: resident refusal, family refusal, cost, and stigma of mental illness were the top four.[15]

Other barriers have presented themselves to me in assisted living facilities; often, merely tracking down the residents is difficult (I once interviewed a resident for 45 minutes in the hair salon while she was under the curling iron). Since most ALFs were conceived and are still marketed as *social environments* geared toward *wellness* (there are few directors of nursing but many wellness directors), they are often ill-suited to residents with dementia. Cocktail hours, "mystery" rides in the facility bus, and resident council meetings are often not appropriate for cognitively impaired residents. Often, facility resources are directed toward marketing staff, leaving a noticeable absence of social work staff. The facility medical charts are often mere fragments of what I've come to expect from nursing homes, with rare detailed medical or social histories and minimal documentation of residents' mood and behavior problems. Some facilities are so opposed to being perceived as health care institutions that they actually forbid the use of formal charts in their buildings.

Often (but not always), even the resident is unable to provide a reliable history, so I attempt to contact a family member to provide information. If I'm successful, I have to keep my radar up for signs of biased information. For example, the family may be reluctant to disclose problematic behaviors preceding admission for fear of their loved one being asked to leave. Financial pressures (most residents are private pay) often lead to questionable decisions, such as insisting the resident is capable of reliably taking his or her own medications to avoid the extra monthly fee for having the assistance of the nurse or medical technician. In fact, the recent severe recession has impacted those in assisted living much more than those in nursing homes, who have typically already "spent down" their assets to qualify for Medicaid. Finally, family members may become defensive and resentful when they learn that "the psychiatrist" has been asked to see their loved one, fearing a dementia diagnosis and its implications.

Many states now have enhanced standards for the care of residents with dementia, with Massachusetts creating a new Special Care Residence certification category and Florida now requiring facilities to monitor and manage ALF residents who wander. In fact, wandering and elopement are serious problems in assisted living facilities. Unlike a couple that runs away to get married, elopement from assisted living facilities by residents with Alzheimer's disease and other dementias is a growing problem. Traditionally defined as leaving a locked or secure psychiatric institution without notice or permission, the term has expanded to refer to the many residents of nursing homes, assisted living facilities, and other types of senior housing who wander away or leave secure dementia units without permission. Up to 60 percent of people with dementia will wander at least once, and there are many causes of wandering in dementia. Facilities need to consider precautionary measures to decrease the risk of elopements, including alarms, wrist bands, signs warning visitors of the risk, monitored exit doors, and even having high-risk residents move to rooms that allow for closer staff supervision.

Finally, I'd like to comment on a recent trend in ALFs, that of incorporating or later adding a "secure dementia unit" in the facility. In fact, one-third of providers polled in a recent study operate combined ALF/dementia care residences. Twenty-four states require facilities to disclose, often in writing, the attributes that make their special care units different from other parts of the facility. To minimize stigma, these units often have soothing names, such as Willows, Bridges, or Life Guidance. While often well intentioned, these units may be plagued by problems. Many are understaffed and have a lack of commitment to true staff education, serious activities programming, and clear-cut criteria related to when nursing home placement is necessary. Imagine how devastating it is for a person with mild dementia to find himself or herself "locked up," unable to even venture outside for a walk without special arrangements being made. Residents have made impassioned pleas to me to end what they view as their incarceration, their imprisonment, their near complete loss of freedom. Few exercises are as futile in dementia care as trying to explain to someone with Alzheimer's disease why he or she needs to be in a secure unit. At best, you can keep your words simple and try to be as calm and reassuring as possible. These are of course some of the most difficult conversations to have with someone who requires the security of a special care unit but who can't accept or understand it. While aging in place (not having to move from one's present residence to receive care or services as one ages) is a central tenet of the ALF philosophy, the reality is that there are often no clear-cut criteria regarding the level of functional disability or illness that residents may have while in a facility. This problem cuts both ways; I've been involved in several cases where the state has stepped in to argue that nursing home transfer is indicated as a result of advanced dementia, yet I disagreed with their opinion and advocated for the resident to remain where they were. In my opinion, these should be case-by-case decisions and driven by function and safety issues rather than solely by scores on dementia screening tests.

Some ALF critics argue that facilities have too much discretion over the discharge of residents, while others suggest that facilities are overly aggressive in admitting residents that have issues and needs that are beyond the facilities' capabilities. While both sides have valid arguments, in my experience the latter criticism is most valid. Marketing staff are prized and highly influential, often trumping the clinical staff in decisions to admit residents to settings that can't possibly meet the challenges and demands that these residents present. As with the nursing home environment described in Chapter 1 dementia has now pervaded the assisted living industry, wreaking havoc on staff, families, and residents alike.

Let's review additional "reality lessons" learned about assisted living facilities, and the practical strategies that can be used when this situation becomes an option for you and your loved one. Keep in mind that many of the strategies in Chapter 4 are still applicable here.

LESSON 1: SUPERIOR AESTHETICS AND HIGH-END PERKS

Strategies

1. Don't be taken in so much by the beauty and amenities: when it comes to dementia, the presence of caring, well-trained staff; supervised activities; smart design features; and attention to resident safety are far more important. If you move your loved one into a facility, alert the staff of any prior history of wandering or elopement attempts at other facilities.
2. Inquire about the presence of dementia-relevant services: cognitive and psychiatric assessments as well as therapy and social work services.

LESSON 2: VARYING STATE REGULATIONS

Strategy

Research how your state regulates ALFs. The National Center for Assisted Living's 2011 Assisted Living State Regulatory Review offers a state-by-state summary of assisted living regulations covering 21 categories. It is available for free download.[16]

LESSON 3: AGING IN PLACE PHILOSOPHY

Strategies

1. Inquire what the facility's policy and culture is about mandatory nursing home placement if and when dementia progresses. Are hospice and/or palliative services available on-site? While many residents and families don't want to leave assisted living once they have experienced the benefits, realize that many ALFs are not able to handle the skilled care needs required in advanced dementia.
2. Ask if companions or other professional staff hired privately may be brought in to supplement facility staff on a case-by-case basis.

LESSON 4: QUESTIONS TO ASK IN YOUR SEARCH FOR AN ASSISTED LIVING FACILITY

Strategy

Once you've determined that assisted living is the right setting for your loved one, you need to think about the factors that are important in deciding on one or another facility. They should include the staff's expertise and awareness of Alzheimer's disease, and the ability of the staff to meet your loved one's medical and medication needs. Here are five essential questions to ask:

1. What specific education and training do the staff receive in dementia care?
2. What activities are available, and are they supervised?
3. What is the availability of cognitive and psychiatric assessments in your facility?
4. What is your facility's policy and culture around transfer to a nursing home as my loved one's dementia worsens?
5. Which staff will administer medications, and how are medical problems handled when they arise?

LESSON 5: PAYING FOR AN ASSISTED LIVING FACILITY

Strategy

Unlike for nursing homes, government financial assistance for ALFs is very limited. Average costs are approximately $2,800/month, and about a third of ALFs charge a one-time entrance fee. While 40 percent of ALF residents pay for services themselves, nearly half use family funds to pay. After self-pay and family support, Medicaid is the next largest source of payment. More than 40 states cover services for qualified, low-income people through Medicaid waiver programs. Waivers were created primarily so that people who would have otherwise had to go to a nursing home are able to live in an ALF instead.

Here are five essential questions to ask about ALF costs:

1. What is included in the basic fee, and what extra fees are charged?
2. When and how often are rates increased?
3. What is the refund policy?
4. What are my options if and when our funds are depleted?
5. What happens if my loved one's medical needs increase or the level of care changes? Foe example, your loved one may be able to give herself a shower and take her own medications now, but a year from now that may change.

6

RESPITE CARE: MORE THAN JUST A BREAK

Receiving temporary relief from the stresses of caregiving for a loved one with Alzheimer's disease (AD) cannot be overemphasized as a positive experience for both the caregiver and the person with dementia. While many people derive great satisfaction and self-esteem from their role as caregiver, we have seen in Chapter 3 that the toll is enormous. Without temporary breaks from caregiving, a person will undoubtedly face burnout: anxiety, anger, irritability, resentfulness, even extreme fatigue and serious health problems like ulcers, migraines, and high blood pressure. This chapter will review the primary respite care options available to dementia caregivers: adult day care, home health care aides, and geriatric care managers.

ADULT DAY SERVICES

According to the National Adult Day Services Association, there are currently more than 4,600 adult day centers in the United States that service more than 260,000 participants and their caregivers. The increasing flexibility and convenience of these programs for people with Alzheimer's disease makes them true godsends for thousands of caregivers, not to mention terrific sources of mental and social stimulation for people with dementia. Let's take a closer look at what these programs actually are before we decide how we are going to entice our loved one to go.

Generally speaking, adult day care is a planned program of activities that may be appropriate for people in very mild to even moderately severe stages of Alzheimer's disease. Most operate during daytime hours Monday through Friday, although increasingly programs are offering weekend and evening hours. These programs have existed for over 30 years but only recently have

grown rapidly. California, Texas, and Pennsylvania have more than 200 programs each, and 11 other states have between 100 and 200 programs. Much
like assisted living, these centers are regulated by the states, and states use
guidelines, licensure, and/or certification to ensure compliance.[1]

For people with dementia, an ideal ratio of staff to participants is four to one,
and most programs operate with a director, a social worker, activities staff,
personal care aides, and a registered or licensed practical nurse. Some may even
have close working relationships with pharmacists and geriatricians who
provide medical and medication management oversight.

More than 60 percent of adult day centers provide the following services:
meals, therapeutic activities (games, walks, excursions, art and music), personal
assistance, social services, health-related services, medication management,
transportation, personal care services, and caregiver support groups. Some provide rehabilitation therapy, exercises, advice about home safety, and even individual and group counseling. Some centers even offer programs that include
children. For example, some centers offer intergenerational programs in which
children and older adults who are attending separate day programs in the same
location have opportunities to be in contact with each other.

People who seem to benefit the most from adult day centers are those who
are in the earlier stages of dementia, those who enjoy opportunities for socializ-
ing and making new friendships, and those who don't require 24-hour supervision. Centers that are designed specifically for people with dementia may also
help those beyond the mild stage of illness.

Unfortunately, the reality is that getting a person to agree to go is often the
biggest challenge. Much like getting a hard-of-hearing older person to agree to
a hearing aid, enticing an older person to go to an adult day program may be
similarly difficult. Common excuses I hear from people who seem like they
would benefit from such an environment include:

1. Those places are just not for me.
2. I don't want to be with old people all day.
3. The next stop after this is the nursing home.

Tackling those excuses head on is often the best strategy. If the caregiver
doesn't believe adult day services are worth pursuing, it's not likely to happen.
Often a short initial visit at a time when an activity the person with dementia
might actually enjoy is going on is a terrific way to get things started. Just one
or two visits per week may be the way to go early on, with more days added
when things get more comfortable and routinized. These programs work best
for people who want to be there, so it's important for them to see for themselves
that an adult day program may be a positive way to spend a few hours a day.

The cost of adult day programs is typically reasonable. The average cost of
adult day care is $67 per day, which includes meals and/or snacks. Some cen-
ters offer financial assistance through grants or government contracts, and in

some cases Medicaid pays for it. Many centers offer services on a sliding scale so that cost varies based on income and ability to pay.

In-Home Respite Care

Having breaks while their loved ones receive supervision and social interaction in their own homes can be incredibly beneficial for caregivers.

Home care has changed dramatically over the years, with more than 20,000 home care agencies now operating in the United States. When the Medicare program started in 1965, home health services were limited to people who were acutely ill; home health services had to be deemed medically necessary. People with dementia and other chronic illnesses were expected to get help from informal caregivers, not the nurses, aides, and other providers who make up the home health agencies (HHAs) of today. In the 1990s, the interpretation of home care benefits changed, and providers took advantage of the opportunity to serve a more diverse home care population with chronic illnesses like dementia. By 2001, the number of Medicare-certified HHAs was 6,861, and the number climbed to 8,618 in 2006. More than 3 million people received Medicare-financed home health care in 2005.[2]

In addition to Medicare-certified HHAs, home care is also provided through home care aide organizations, visiting nurse associations, and hospices. Thousands of agencies provide care that is not certified by Medicare, and each state has different licensing and oversight requirements.

Most people with or without dementia have an intense desire to remain in their homes as long as possible. When combined with the government's growing desire to shift care of seniors from institutions to community-based settings, there have never been more opportunities for caregivers to find home care assistance. To that end, caregivers of people with Alzheimer's disease looking for both respite care and in-home assistance have several choices when it comes to finding a home care aide.

Volunteer home care aides provide companionship, supervision, and sometimes light meal preparation. Although they normally can't provide personal care like bathroom assistance and grooming, the fact that they are free and often very dedicated make them potentially invaluable to family caregivers who need some respite. Community organizations and religious groups are places to look for volunteer home care aides, as is a nationwide volunteer program called the Senior Companion Program.

Private home care aides are typically self-employed and not associated with any agency. Many of these aides are found through ads in local papers or word of mouth. Compared to aides that are sent by an agency, an advantage here is that the caregiver has more control over who is hired and the services provided. Private aides are generally willing to provide any kind of care needed, including personal care such as bathroom assistance and bathing, but the caregiver needs to ensure the aide is qualified to perform these tasks. Many caregivers don't have the time or confidence to check references and employment history of potential aides, and private home care is generally not covered by insurance. Keeping financial records of these arrangements is a must. I've met many terrific private home care aides who had previously worked in nursing homes or assisted living facilities, and when the fit is a good one, there is no question of the value of the aide to the caregiver and the person with dementia.

The third option for finding home care aides is the most common: home care agencies. The agencies are helpful because they ensure aides are trained and have passed background and reference checks, and they also do the bookkeeping and recordkeeping. Depending on the agency, aides can perform certain medical procedures. Disadvantages of agency aides include having less control over who is sent to the caregiver's home as well as costs that are often higher than private home care aides. Agencies do sometimes accept private health insurance or government assistance, and they are easily found in the phone book under home health services or via Internet search engines. Interestingly, while typical long-term care insurance policies offer benefits for a combination of nursing home care, assisted living care, and home care, consumers can also purchase home-care-only policies. These policies may cover adult day programs along with home health care.

When it comes to Alzheimer's disease and other dementias, home care aides run the gamut in terms of training, experience, and interpersonal skills. Being gentle but firm when it comes to redirection and distraction, speaking calmly but slowly, and encouraging activities that are well suited to the person with dementia are skills that aren't acquired automatically. Some aides work better with people with chronic medical problems than with people with cognitive problems. It's possible to receive 50 hours of dementia training yet still treat someone with Alzheimer's disease as a child rather than as an adult. In my view, having a sense of humor and helping a person with dementia feel useful and dignified are far more important abilities as a home health aide than knowing that being restless or pacing is a sign of having moderate as opposed to mild dementia.

GERIATRIC CARE MANAGERS

Geriatric care managers are eldercare specialists who are best viewed as experienced guides and resources for families and caregivers of older adults. They may be trained and experienced in any of several fields related to care management, including nursing, social work, gerontology, or psychology. In my experience, they are most often either advanced practice nurses or social workers with masters degrees. Geriatric care managers that are members of the National Association of Professional Geriatric Care Managers (NAPGCM) are committed to adhering to the NAPGCM Code of Ethics and Standards of Practice, both of which may be found on NAPGCM's website.[3]

When it comes to Alzheimer's disease and other dementias, geriatric care managers may be especially helpful in certain respects. Their strengths include the care planning assessments they conduct to identify needs and problems, and then propose solutions, as well as the continuity of care management they provide: they coordinate communications between family members, doctors, and other professionals. They also help with crises, moves to assisted living facilities or nursing homes, and disputes that may arise between family members. Ideally, their efforts pay off in several ways: caregiver stress is reduced, unnecessary hospitalizations are avoided, and the person with dementia receives well-coordinated care.

With the right geriatric care manager and the ability to afford his or her services (they bill in a variety of ways, but typically their hourly rates range from $50 to $200), I have no doubt that in certain circumstances it can be a wise investment. Keep in mind that the average engagement with a geriatric care manager is likely 20 to 40 hours of work, so the total cost can easily climb into the thousands of dollars. In addition to really understanding Alzheimer's disease and other dementias, a good geriatric care manager should be knowledgeable about local resources and health care professionals, and have a relatively high level of assertiveness and persistence.

WHEN REMAINING AT HOME IS UNWISE OR UNSAFE

As I mentioned earlier in this chapter, most people with and without dementia have an intense desire to remain at home as long as possible. Unfortunately, the reality is that all too often people with dementia stay in their homes well beyond what is safe and conducive to their quality of life. Sometimes families go to great lengths to ensure home care services are adequate and in place, yet their loved one either refuses to allow these professionals in or is too abusive and agitated to permit them to help.

There is no easy answer to the question of when it is time to move a person with dementia from his or her home. It is often a heart-wrenching decision, one in which the caregiver feels guilty, defeated, and inadequate. Each family must take into account how severe their loved one's illness is, as well as their own ability to cope with the effects of the illness on their own lives. While respite options like adult day care and home health aides are often helpful, they can't prevent the inevitability that eventually virtually everyone with dementia requires institutional care. One important factor in this decision is of course the person's safety in their home.

HOME SAFETY AND ALZHEIMER'S DISEASE

Paying attention to safety issues may help delay the need for long-term care for a person with dementia. Paying attention to lighting, for example, may help prevent falls. Particular hazards include stairs and dimly lit corridors. Wearing shoes with rubber soles may help avoid slipping, and loose floor tiles or frayed carpets are disasters waiting to happen. Appliances are notorious for their dangers when people with Alzheimer's disease forget to turn them off. Kettles, for example, should have automatic cut-off switches for when they are turned on and forgotten. Electrical appliances and tools may need to be secured, and thermostatic temperature regulators may be installed for the bath or shower.

WANDERING IN ALZHEIMER'S DISEASE

By far the most serious home safety hazard for a person with dementia is wandering. It's estimated that up to two-thirds of people with Alzheimer's disease in the United States will wander at least once from their home or their caregiver. Wandering occurs at all stages of Alzheimer's disease and in all places where people with dementia live: home, assisted living facilities, and even nursing homes. Facilities need to consider precautionary measures to decrease chances of dangerous wandering, including alarms, wrist bands, signs warning visitors of the risk, monitored exit doors, and even moving high-risk residents to rooms that allow for closer staff supervision.

As with most dementia-related behavioral problems, wandering has many possible causes in Alzheimer's disease. It may be a way of expressing anxiety or agitation, or it may be a response to something as simple as misinterpreting what's going on in the environment. An increasingly common cause of wandering seems to be a desire to fulfill former obligations and tasks. On May 5, 2010, the *New York Times* ran a front-page story on wandering in dementia. In Oregon, for example, the number of searches for lost male Alzheimer's patients nearly doubled from 2008 to 2009. In Arizona, people with dementia have been known to "simply stride out into the desert in high summer and vanish." The article emphasized the importance of learning about the wanderer's life story, for example, work and military history. One man in Virginia who was a former dairy farmer was lost for days after he headed to a local cow pasture, believing it was time for the morning milking. World War II veterans have been known to go long distances, believing they needed to report to base or the front lines.[4]

As with many aspects of dementia care, ingenuity and technology are playing more important roles when it comes to wandering. One caregiver disguised his home's doors with posters that look like bookshelves, and a family hid their loved one's baseball caps since he wouldn't leave the house without wearing one. Technology is also helping, as more companies that make Global Positioning System (GPS) devices have entered the Alzheimer's market. For example, the Alzheimer's Association has a service called Comfort Zone, which is a Web-based GPS location management service that tracks the location of a person with Alzheimer's disease and alerts caregivers when their loved one has migrated out of their predetermined "comfort zone."[5] A service called

EmFinders is another community solution to the problem of wandering. EmFinders uses cellphone technology to determine the exact location of a specially designed device that is worn by the person with Alzheimer's.[6] Finally, the LoJack Corporation recently introduced LoJack Safety Net, a rescue system in which the person with Alzheimer's is outfitted with a bracelet on his or her wrist or ankle. The bracelet constantly emits a radio frequency signal that can be tracked by law enforcement. These signals can be tracked regardless of where the person has wandered, including bodies of water, wooded areas, and steel buildings.[7]

Before moving on to look more closely at inpatient psychiatric units, let's analyze some of the most useful strategies and ideas related to adult day centers and prevention of wandering.

LESSON 1: TIPS FOR CHOOSING AN ADULT DAY CENTER

Strategies

1. Spend some time at one or two centers you're considering to get a feel for the staff, the other residents, and the environment.
2. Ask questions about staffing, licensure, activities, services provided, and costs. Do they seem to offer programs that appeal to your loved one, whether individually or in groups? Do they seem savvy about working with people with dementia?
3. Be honest with staff about your loved one's interests, personality quirks, and propensity to get agitated or upset in certain situations. A good fit is essential to success.

LESSON 2: STEPS TO TAKE FOR PREVENTION OF WANDERING

Strategies

1. Consider placing darkly colored mats by exit doors, and consider painting exit doors the same color as the walls to camouflage them.
2. Consider installing warning alarms on exit doors so that you will be able to respond quickly and at any hour of the day or night.
3. Consider discreetly labeling your loved one's clothing with a telephone number.
4. Consider enrolling your loved one in MedicAlert + Alzheimer's Association Safe Return, a 24-hour nationwide emergency response service for individuals with Alzheimer's or a related dementia who wander or have a medical emergency.[8]

7

THE INPATIENT PSYCHIATRIC UNIT: ALL THOSE RESOURCES BUT SO LITTLE TIME

Psychiatric inpatient hospitals have come a long way since the days they were called asylums or institutions for the insane. Thanks to more effective medications and the shifting of older people from psychiatric hospitals to nursing homes in the 1970s, inpatient psychiatry units are no longer major centers for psychiatric care. A key advantage of hospital care for people with dementia is that the intensive nature of this setting allows for a more thorough opportunity to "get to the bottom" of the problem that necessitated admission in the first place. An unexpected disadvantage, as we'll explore, is that easy availability of specialized hospital care for people with dementia-related behavioral problems may lead to overutilization of these settings as a respite stay for stressed caregivers and long-term care facility staff.

In theory, the primary role of the inpatient psychiatric unit for the person with dementia is to stabilize an acute situation when behavioral problems become dangerous or life threatening. Consider, for example, a nursing home resident who has become increasingly combative, other residents are at risk, and the decision is made to transport the resident to the area hospital that has a geriatric psychiatry inpatient unit and an available bed. The rules are different here: patients can be involuntarily committed, intramuscular (IM) medications for acute agitation and aggression are more widely administered, and physical restraints are viewed more permissively.

The general idea is that here virtually all resources are available: round-the-clock behavioral monitoring by trained, experienced psychiatric staff; daily rounds by the psychiatrist; and access to consultations by neurologists and internists or geriatricians. Neuropsychological testing may be done to provide further diagnostic clarification and guide future interventions. Occupational and physical therapy are available, as are seasoned social workers and case managers who can help to involve family members in the treatment process and to navigate the complicated array of financial issues and community resources. Daily activities may include exercise, music therapy, bright light therapy, and therapeutic groups. Existing psychiatric medications can be tapered and stopped to establish a current baseline of symptoms, and new medications can be introduced with close monitoring of side effects and efficacy. Ideally, communication with the nursing home and past providers takes place, ensuring that everyone involved is "on the same page" and a true multidisciplinary team effort occurs.

REASONS FOR ADMISSION

Let's look at the reasons an elderly person with dementia might get admitted to an inpatient psychiatric unit. Far and away the number one reason is the person's behavior. Physical aggression that includes combative, assaultive behaviors is much more common than the other behavioral precipitants of psychiatric admission, while wandering and attempting to elope from home or a facility is usually the next most common reason. Verbal agitation and aggression such as screaming, threatening others, or insulting others may precipitate admission. Displaying sexually inappropriate behaviors is another trigger for inpatient admission, especially if other vulnerable residents with dementia are being victimized. Behaviors considered self-endangering may lead to inpatient admission, including being unable to care for oneself, living in squalor, refusing medications, and refusing assistance to the point of dangerousness. I'll never forget the time an elderly gentleman living in his own home was admitted after the water meter reader alerted authorities that he was crawling to answer the door (he could no longer walk). Other reasons for a person with dementia to be admitted to a psychiatric inpatient unit include severe depression, anxiety, paranoia, mania, or other underlying psychiatric symptom.

LENGTH OF STAY

Compared with the mid 1990s when I completed my fellowship training in geriatric psychiatry, average lengths of stay on these hospital units have declined considerably, to approximately 8 to 10 days from well over 20. Consider the following recent description of the geriatric inpatient psychiatry unit at McLean Hospital in Belmont, Massachusetts, a Harvard Medical School affiliate.

Geriatric Psychiatry Unit[1]

The geriatric psychiatry unit is a short-term, inpatient unit for the evaluation and treatment of adults, usually age 60 years or older, with disorders of cognitive functioning, mood, or reality testing that are often accompanied by medical disorders. The unit treats a range of psychiatric conditions in the elderly and has special expertise in treating Alzheimer's disease (AD) and other forms of dementia. The medical, nursing, and other staff of the geriatric psychiatry unit are experts in evaluating patients with mild to severe dementia and in separating those behavioral and emotional problems that are dementia-related from those that are due to other causes that may require specific treatment interventions. The geriatric psychiatry unit uses an intensive multidisciplinary approach that integrates behavioral interventions, therapeutic milieu, psychopharmacology, and other somatic approaches to stabilize patients rapidly and implement treatment plans that maximize cognitive and emotional functioning in patients and thus enhance their quality of life.

Having treated elderly patients in four different geriatric psychiatry inpatient units since completion of my fellowship in 1996, I wonder how much can realistically be accomplished for some of these complicated patients in such a brief period of time. Because the hospital environment is so drastically different from the nursing home or ALF environment (the hospital is more controlled, structured, with generally better trained and more experienced staff), the behaviors that were occurring in the facility often do not manifest themselves in the hospital. For example, physical aggression in a person with dementia is often precipitated by a specific situation or provocation. Feeling *overwhelmed* by tasks that are too demanding, *overstimulated* by noises or activities, or *frightened* by unfamiliar people may trigger verbal or physical aggression. These "catastrophic reactions" are best managed by prevention: stopping them before they happen by anticipating the environmental triggers. An intervention as simple as switching the seating arrangement in the dining room of the assisted living facility or nursing home may do the trick. But once the patient arrives at the hospital, these triggers are no longer present, and the behaviors often don't occur.

This leads to the dilemma of expecting the psychiatrist in the hospital to alter a medication regimen without observing the behaviors that were reported to have occurred. Changing medications based solely on reports of others is very difficult for most psychiatrists to do, and therefore the same medications are frequently continued, often leading to recurrence of the behaviors on return to the facility, where the maladaptive patterns in the environment repeat themselves. Most psychiatrists and other hospital staff who work on inpatient psychiatric units don't also work in nursing homes or assisted living facilities and don't really understand the issues and obstacles that these facilities face. They may tell themselves, "Well, if the patient is calm and pleasant here, there's no reason he shouldn't be calm and pleasant at the nursing home too." They also usually don't have any motivation or incentive to reach out to the nursing home and other out-of-hospital providers for detailed records and descriptions of actual incidents that led to the hospitalization in the first place. Hospitals often work too independently; they insulate themselves from the outside provider community for a whole host of reasons. Hospital psychiatrists have their hospital's internal rules and regulations to attend to, pressures to meet productivity goals, and other interests and projects. Their success and pride don't typically stem from how well patients do back in their long-term care environments. The hospitalization is merely a brief respite for the nursing home staff (if the patient returns to that same facility) or an opportunity for the nursing home to balk at the patient returning, arguing that they "can no longer meet his needs."

It's not just psychiatric hospitalizations that occur too often in people with dementia, but medical hospitalizations as well. In a study published in the *New England Journal of Medicine* in September 2011, researchers examined Medicare data involving almost 475,000 patients with "advanced mental and functional impairments who were in a nursing home at least 120 days before their deaths." Among these patients, 19% were sent to hospitals or other nursing homes for questionable reasons in their final months, often ending up up in intensive care or with feeding tubes. Rates of such transfers differed widely between states: from 2 percent in Alaska to 37 percent in Louisiana.

When asked whether she thought money might be a motivating factor for these transfers, (Medicare pays three times the normal daily rate for nursing homes to take patients back after a brief hospitalization) Joan Teno, MD, a palliative care physician and coauthor of the study, commented, "I think that's unfortunately a factor in what's happening here. A lot of this care just feels like in and out, in and out. You really have to question, is the health care system doing a good job or not."[2]

I've seen the same resident in six different nursing homes, with the cycle of hospitalization and refusal of the nursing home to accept the resident back repeating itself multiple times. Of course, there *are* those truly refractory patients whose behaviors are so problematic that they really don't belong in *any* nursing home: unfortunately, the dwindling number of state hospital beds throughout the country makes state hospitalization unrealistic as well. Keep in mind that these observations are largely based on experience as well as informal discussions with peers; there are no data available that I am aware of that shed light on these issues in a formal manner. In Rhode Island, the variability in rates of nursing home transfers to psychiatric inpatient units is high: one nursing home with 150 beds had over 60 hospital admissions for psychiatric issues in 2007, while others had none or one. Even factoring in the differences in the medical and behavioral complexity of the residents, the variability is in part due to the *subjective* nature of the decision-making process. From one home to another, directors of nursing and administrators have different thresholds for tolerating aggression and other psychiatric symptoms.

Other factors that inevitably color these decisions are the extent to which the resident's family is "difficult," the current census and waiting list of the transferring facility, and the role of the attending physician and psychiatric provider in the facility. Not surprisingly, medicolegal concerns also play a role here; if a resident threatens suicide or harm to another resident, some administrators feel they *must* send the resident out to an emergency department for "clearance" to return to the facility. Unfortunately, these situations are often handled poorly and inefficiently; the unpleasant and costly five-hour marathon emergency department visit could have been avoided with some smart questioning of the resident, involvement of family, and appraisal of the real risks and benefits of other actions that could be taken (medication adjustment, closer staff supervision of the resident for a specified time period, telephone consultation with the psychiatric provider, etc.).

The call to 911 happens all too often in long-term care facilities, whether from an assisted living resident with mild dementia and paranoia who's convinced her wallet has just been stolen or from the charge nurse in the nursing home who panics when a male resident with dementia touches a female resident inappropriately.

In my opinion, involving police in dementia cases is not the best use of law enforcement resources: they are usually poorly educated about dementia, and their involvement in dementia-related behavioral problems sends the wrong message, that on some level these behaviors rise to the level of criminality. In the nursing home murder case described in Chapter 4 in which I was involved as an expert witness, the perpetrator, who clearly suffered from at least moderately severe dementia, was to be tried for murder in criminal court. Only after he was found to be incompetent to stand trial was he involuntarily hospitalized as opposed to jailed. A more common scenario, that of an 86-year-old woman with mild dementia who in March 2009 at 3 A.M. wandered from her senior citizen complex, illustrates the lack of dementia education found in most police departments. The taxi driver who was called by a local gas station attendant to take her home instead brought her to a police precinct when she couldn't tell him her address. According to her family, officers went through her bag, found her address, and instructed the cab driver to take her home. Only after she arrived back at the senior citizen complex with no keys did the cab driver locate an emergency contact card in her bag, enabling him to call her daughter and notify her of the incident. Her daughter commented, "If it had not been for the cab driver, I would not have been aware of this incident . . . it could have continued." For their part, the police acknowledged they do not have a policy "specifically dealing with Alzheimer's patients."[3]

VERBAL AGITATION: YELLING AND SCREAMING

In my experience, a recurring clinical example of the *inappropriate* use of an inpatient psychiatric hospitalization is for a person with dementia who is exhibiting a form of severe verbal agitation most people would refer to as yelling or screaming. While medical jargon may characterize it as "dementia-related pathological yelling," "vocally disruptive behavior," or "noisemaking," essentially we are referring to a person who is loud and disruptive to others. In some ways, it is a cruel irony that a symptom seemingly so simple and easy to describe is so difficult to treat. Consider the following case, which is not particularly unusual, described in an August 2008 letter in the *Journal of Neuropsychiatry and Clinical Neurosciences*:

> Ms. A is an 88-year-old woman with no previous psychiatric admissions and a 6-year history of probable Alzheimer's disease dementia and Parkinson's disease. She was transferred to the medical psychiatry unit from a nursing facility for treatment of behavioral dyscontrol. She exhibited 2 months of increasing verbal agitation in the form of screaming, hollering obscenities, and pallilalia [i.e., repeating words rapidly and involuntarily]. Her screaming periods would last over 45 minutes, several times daily, and she was unresponsive to comfort measures or reassurance. Two months prior to admission she was treated with risperidone and then quetiapine with no improvement. A trial of escitalopram was ineffective. Subsequent trials of olanzapine and divalproex were similarly ineffective.[4]

The case description proceeds to describe noticeable improvement after 11 electroconvulsive therapy (ECT) treatments, as "the staff noticed marked changes in her verbal behavior by the second ECT treatment when she looked at a peer and spoke in grammatically correct sentences at normal volume. She began to socialize with visitors without verbal agitation."

My point in presenting this case is not to endorse ECT as the preferred treatment for yelling behaviors, but rather to illustrate how common yet poorly responsive to medications these behaviors tend to be. Furthermore, there has been little written about these behaviors in the dementia literature. Consider the following, from Part 1 of the excellent piece "Screaming and Wailing in Dementia Patients," by Bernard Groulx, MD, CM, FRCPC:

> While screaming is a major concern for everyone working in the field of dementia, there have been very few studies on this behaviour specifically, and even less attention has been given to the topic in academic literature. For example, the academic book I consider to be the best resource on Alzheimer's Disease (AD) and recommend for everyone in the field of AD management, entitled *Clinical Diagnosis and Management of Alzheimer's Disease*, has only a little over 30 words on the subject of screaming.[5]

Reasons cited to explain screaming in dementia are many, and thorough clinicians will try to explore all in their search for answers: pain, constipation, hunger, thirst, overstimulation, understimulation, recent room change, fear, loneliness, depression, and psychosis.

Typically, persons exhibiting these behaviors will get switched from one medication to another in the nursing home without noticeable improvement, until the disturbances in the facility are so great that in desperation a psychiatric admission is sought. Instead, what's called for are creative and imaginative attempts at solutions that may include medications but don't rely on them exclusively. Even periodically using a soundproof booth or room is a preferable alternative to hospitalization in many cases. In the book *Clinical Diagnosis and*

Management of Alzheimer's Disease, Rubin Becker and James Lindesay write, "Some rooms should have sound proofing capabilities to accommodate noisy patients."[6]

Another factor that is worth keeping in mind is the profitability of these inpatient units to the hospitals themselves. Consider why geropsych units are so popular. In the FAQ section of the Behavioral Health Concepts, Inc. website, the following answer is provided:

> Geropsych Units are very popular because of two primary factors. Demographics show a growing and aging, underserved population. Most mental health problems of the elderly are attributed to the aging process rather than a unique and treatable problem. The second reason is the utilization of unused capacity within the hospital which can also provide an appropriate financial return.[7]

GENERAL HOSPITAL UNIT OR GERIATRIC UNIT?

Another important consideration when it comes to inpatient psychiatric hospitals for the elderly is whether there is a difference in clinical treatment between *general psychiatry* inpatient units and *geriatric psychiatry* inpatient units. Since the emergence of geriatric psychiatry as an organized subspecialty within psychiatry, enough evidence-based clinical knowledge of the elderly has emerged to truly foster better outcomes. Although many studies examining "special care units" for dementia in long-term care facilities have failed to show significant benefit, one study comparing several treatment measures of elderly psychiatric inpatients hospitalized on a specialized geriatric psychiatry inpatient unit compared with elderly psychiatric inpatients on a general psychiatry unit *in the same hospital* did show some distinct advantages. The study showed that compared with similar patients on the general psychiatry unit, a greater percentage of the geriatric psychiatry unit inpatients received complete organic medical workups, structured cognitive assessments, and close monitoring of medication side effects.[8]

These results are not surprising when one considers that these are the themes that are emphasized in geriatric psychiatry fellowships. Unfortunately, as will be explained more fully in chapter 10, the need for geriatric psychiatrists exceeds the supply, and general psychiatrists, nurse practitioners, clinical nurse specialists, and physician assistants will increasingly play a vital role in geriatric mental health service delivery.

While the inpatient psychiatric hospital experience certainly has its flaws, it is nevertheless an important aspect of dementia treatment in the United States. Despite the problems, I've been involved in many cases with successful outcomes, with medication changes leading to symptom stabilization and/or improvement for months or even years after the admission. Some examples of appropriate uses of the hospital for people with dementia include evaluating a person for the use of electroconvulsive therapy and beginning a patient on certain medications that require close monitoring. Clozapine (Clozaril), for example, is an antipsychotic medication that requires blood monitoring and carries multiple warnings for adverse events. While data is lacking to quantify these examples of treatment successes, I believe it is safe to say they are all too infrequent.

Let's now summarize the key themes presented in this chapter and the strategies for caregivers to ensure the inpatient setting is utilized to its maximum advantage.

LESSON 1: INPATIENT PSYCHIATRIC HOSPITALIZATIONS ARE USUALLY OF SHORT DURATION

Strategies

1. Understand and try to agree on the *goals* of the admission. Possibilities may include establishing new medication regimens, developing nonpharmacologic strategies that may be more effective, clarifying diagnosis and prognosis, and assessing for appropriateness of electroconvulsive therapy (ECT).
2. Ensure *communication* occurs between inpatient providers and transferring facility or outpatient providers. For example, if the admission was precipitated by an aggressive episode in the nursing home, ensure that the circumstances and details of the episode are clear and communicated well.

LESSON 2: THE BEHAVIORS THAT LED TO THE HOSPITALIZATION MAY NOT OCCUR IN THE HOSPITAL

Strategies

1. If a goal is changing medications, encourage the treatment team to do so even if the preadmission behaviors don't occur in the hospital
2. Again, ensure *communication* occurs between inpatient providers and transferring facility or outpatient providers.
3. Realize that in addition to medications, there really are interventions not involving medications that have benefit in treating agitation in dementia. These include caregiver education and support, music therapy, behavior management therapies (by professionals), and staff training and education.

LESSON 3: THINK THROUGH IN ADVANCE YOUR FEELINGS ABOUT PSYCHIATRIC INPATIENT ADMISSION

Strategies

1. If you are your loved one's health care proxy, power of attorney, or legal guardian, you really do have a say in the matter. Let the nursing home or assisted living facility know your opinion about the prospect of inpatient psychiatric treatment for your loved one. Specify which (if any) hospital has your preferred

inpatient unit, and recommend alternatives if you do not desire this type of treatment. For example, other options often include medication changes, behavior management strategies, transfer to another long-term care facility, or an opinion from a geriatric psychiatrist.

2. If your loved one does get admitted to an inpatient psychiatric unit, don't passively wait until they return home or back to their previous facility. Communicate with the inpatient treatment team (usually led by a social worker or case manager), expressing your views about what drives your loved one's behavior problems and what interventions have helped in the past.

8

MEMORY CLINICS AND CLINICAL RESEARCH TRIALS: TREATMENT VS. RECRUITMENT

In the fragmented and chaotic world of dementia care, what could sound better than a memory clinic or memory center? Think about it, a place to bring your loved one for comprehensive assessment, treatment planning, medication management, state-of the-art imaging, cerebrospinal fluid analysis, and both neuropsychological and genetic testing. They may even throw in counseling (for both patient and caregiver), education, access to community resources, and invitations to participate in clinical trials. Compared to a rushed primary care physician who may have five minutes (on a good day) to deal with a memory disorder, what an honor and a privilege to be treated with such attention and respect. To many well-educated laypersons who have bought into the notion that excellent treatment is synonymous with the latest sophisticated technology, imagine the appeal of access to accomplished researchers, nuclear medicine imaging techniques such as Single-Photon Emission Computed Tomography (SPECT) and Positron Emission Tomography (PET), and perhaps even the latest innovation in Alzheimer's imaging, the PET imaging of amyloid itself (accumulated protein fragments; one of the hallmarks of Alzheimer's disease [AD]) using the Pittsburgh Compound B (PiB).

Let's begin by exploring the history of memory clinics. James Lindesay nicely summarizes this history.[1] The first memory clinics were set up in the United States in the mid-1970s, aiming to attract patients in the earlier stages of illness. Although they provided assessment, treatment, and advice, from the outset there was an explicit focus on research, particularly treatment trials. They were called memory clinics to avoid the stigma of the word "dementia," and they were usually set up in academic medical centers by professionals with particular research and educational interests. In fact, today the National Institute on Aging funds Alzheimer's Disease Centers at major medical institutions throughout the

United States (a full listing can found at http://www.nia.nih.gov/alzheimers/alzheimers-disease-research-centers).

In the United Kingdom, memory clinics first appeared in the mid-1980s, aiming to forestall deterioration by early diagnosis and treatment, identify and treat disorders other than dementia, evaluate new therapeutic agents, and reassure worried people who don't have dementia-related deficits.[2]

That reassurance aspect of memory clinics and even memory screenings is by no means trivial. With all of life's stresses and distractions, including being overscheduled, sleep-deprived, multitasking with mobile phones and iPads, and struggling in a difficult economy, people worry that "memory lapses" are early signs of Alzheimer's disease. Consider, for example, that most people have gone into a room to get something but then forgot what they went in to get. In most cases, these episodes of forgetfulness reflect either normal age-related memory loss, sleep deprivation, or stress. More concerning is the person who later can't remember what he went into the room to get, or even the entire episode of going into the room.

In normal age-related memory loss, there may be worsening attention and concentration, but vocabulary and understanding of relationships between things don't usually change with aging. In Alzheimer's disease, there is an early and profound problem with recent memory that even cueing and context don't help. So if I ask you to remember three words, one of which is "apple," and ask you in three minutes what the three words were, if you have Alzheimer's disease, you won't remember "apple" even if I say, "One was a fruit." If you have Alzheimer's disease, you may not remember the order of things (chronological memory) or who said what (source memory). You may have trouble finding common words (like "watch" or "pen"), and you may not even recall that conversations or events ever took place. Other worrisome signs include being repetitive (and not just for emphasis) and as we've discussed, not realizing you have a memory problem. In Alzheimer's, there may be intrusions on your memory. For example, if I ask you to draw a cube, in a few minutes you may think that I asked you to remember the word "cube."

Although there has never been an explicit description of what a memory clinic is or of how it should function, most are primarily concerned with the *early* assessment and diagnosis of dementia. Therefore, most patients seen in memory clinics will be able to understand the diagnosis and its implications, including making plans for the future. The multidisciplinary team approach is the rule for most memory clinics. As noted by James Lindesay: "A memory clinic cannot function without a core team of a doctor (psychiatrist, physician, neurologist), a nurse, and appropriate clerical and administrative support. Other professionals who may have regular sessional input into a memory clinic include: clinical psychologists/neuropsychologists; speech and language therapists; occupational therapists; and support workers from voluntary sector organizations such as the Alzheimer's Society."[3] Social workers are also usually part of the core team, and pharmacists and dieticians may also be involved. The actual assessment typically includes a thorough review of general medical health and health history, a physical and neurological examination, and a review of medications and medication history. All patients require a full mental health history and mental status examination. Psychological assessments are usually performed by or under the supervision of a clinical psychologist, while more detailed testing with validated measurement instruments is usually performed by a neuropsychologist. Other important aspects of assessment include functional abilities, input of caregivers, and psychosocial situation. Spiritual and religious aspects of health care are often assessed, along with views and experiences with alternative treatments such as aromatherapy, nutritional products, and acupuncture.

Since screening for Alzheimer's disease is an important part of most assessments for memory problems, it's worth exploring the most widely used of these screening tests, the Mini-Mental Status Examination (MMSE). Introduced by Marshall Folstein and others in 1975, the MMSE tests global cognitive function with items assessing orientation, word recall, attention and calculation, language abilities, and visuospatial ability. To assess orientation to time, for example, which accounts for 5 of the 30 total points, the person is asked to state the year, season, day, date, and month. Scores on the MMSE range from 0 to 30, with scores of 25 or higher generally considered normal. Scores of less than 10 generally indicate severe impairment, while scores between 10 and 19 indicate moderate dementia. People with mild Alzheimer's disease tend to score in the 19 to 24 range. However, scores may need to be adjusted or interpreted differently to account for a person's age, level of education, and race or ethnicity.

A recent study has shown that the MMSE can actually *overdiagnose* dementia when the people being assessed are poorly educated. In the 2010 study of 222 people, it was more accurate to ask people to recite the days of the week backward rather then asking them to either count backward from 100 by 7's or spell the word "world" backward. Considering that this single item accounts for 5 of the 30 points of the MMSE, you can see how a person could appear to have dementia when in fact they don't. As one of the authors, Razia Hafiz, MD, noted: "We are from Eastern North Carolina, where we have a lot of illiterate and low-literacy people. We were falsely classifying a lot of people as having dementia."[4]

In my experience, the strengths of most memory clinics lie in the areas of assessment and diagnosis, while some are also strong at education and caregiver support. Quoting again from Lindesay: "The provision of both practical and emotional support to patients and their families is critical at all stages of their journey. Every contact with the memory clinic is an opportunity to give information and support, and to identify and address any new or unmet needs."[5] Other important roles for memory clinics include acting as a liaison with community agencies (such as the Alzheimer's Association), providing education and training to students and other professionals, assisting families with end-of-life issues, arranging for autopsies, and so on. In addition, a more recent promising development in the memory clinic world is teaching strategies to minimize the effects of impaired memory. These "memory training" approaches seem to show some promise in efficacy but again are most relevant for those with mild illness. Assistive technologies are being used to provide support in the areas of recall, safety, communication, and leisure enhancement.

Patients and their families who enroll in memory clinics often become disappointed when they attempt to tackle many of the tough issues addressed in this book: verbal and physical agitation and aggression, delusions and other psychotic symptoms, navigation of the chaotic long-term care system, and caregiver burden and stress.

The United Kingdom has recently become aggressive in proposing to increase the number of its memory clinics, and both the French and English national dementia strategies propose national networks of memory clinic services to foster early diagnosis and intervention. In early 2009, Professor Sube Banerjee, the government's main adviser in its dementia strategy, described dementia in classic blunt medical language characteristic of the British as "a horrible brain disease" that should receive "top priority." He noted that although dementia services around the country varied, in general the level of provision was "vanishingly small." The British government has earmarked approximately $250 million for a five-year strategy that will establish clinics as "one-stop shops," offering "expert assessment, support, information and advice to those with memory problems and their carers." Care Services Minister Phil Hope commented, "If you get early diagnosis and early interventions it improves the patient's quality of life, so we are talking about a major rollout of memory clinics. There will be a memory clinic in every town."[6]

It is estimated in the United Kingdom that two-thirds of people with dementia go undiagnosed. Certainly the British plan is ambitious: school children and employers are to be taught about dementia, dementia advisers will be hired to help patients and their families, and extra training will be provided to help general practitioners "spot dementia warning signs."[7]

Not surprisingly, the reaction to the launch of the United Kingdom dementia strategy has been muted: whether the clinics will be adequately funded, whether restrictions on access to drugs will be lifted, and whether the strategy will form part of a comprehensive strategy of treating the disease are all unanswered questions at this time. In June 2011, after much advocacy in the United Kingdom by supporters and volunteers, the National Institute for Health and Clinical Excellence (NICE) increased access to the Alzheimer's drugs available.

In the Executive Summary of the World Alzheimer Report 2011, it was noted that the growth of memory clinics may be an important factor contributing to early dementia diagnosis. In the Netherlands, where there has been a 5-fold increase in the number of memory clinics over the last 10 years, the estimated percentage of all new cases of dementia diagnosed by the memory clinics has risen from 5 to 27 percent.

Ironically, successfully diagnosing patients early leads to an unfortunate conundrum: the currently approved medications for Alzheimer's disease don't work nearly as well as we would like. Speaking at a *Lancet* conference in London in February 2009, Iain Chalmers, editor of the James Lind Library and formerly of the Cochrane Collaboration, said that he was skeptical about the proposed memory clinics: "People ask why the National Institute for Health and Clinical Excellence (NICE) is limiting access to Alzheimer's drugs. Well, the costs are rising very fast and they are not fantastically good. We are going to all have these memory clinics but what do we do when we diagnose someone?"[8]

Asian countries, many of which severely stigmatize and socially ostracize people with mental illness, are beginning to make great strides in recognizing the disease early, educating the population, and destigmatizing Alzheimer's disease. South Korea, for example, is in the midst of a "war on dementia" that involves not only education and emphasizing early recognition, but also real hands-on experience. Children 11 to 13 years old are taught to do hand and foot massages for nursing home patients with dementia, and educational outreach is provided to bank tellers, bus drivers, hair stylists, and postal workers. In 2009, about $1 billion (US) of government and public insurance money in South Korea was spent on patients with dementia. Still, with the over-65 population expected to jump from 7 percent in 2000 to 20 percent in 2026, dementia is straining the country socially and economically. South Korea's effort appears creative and innovative. Dr. Yang Dong-won, who directs one of the many government-run diagnostic centers in Seoul, has visited kindergartens and has brought tofu. "This is very soft, like the brain," he says, letting it crash down. Now, "The brain is damaged."[9]

In the United States, caution is exercised in translating exciting research findings to clinical practice. In July 2009, a paper concluded that three measurable biomarkers could be used to predict outcomes (i.e., which patients with mild cognitive impairment [MCI] would progress to developing Alzheimer's disease over a two-year period). The authors suggested that these markers may be useful in identifying patients for clinical trials and possibly screening tests in memory clinics.[10]

Biomarkers are biological properties that can be detected and measured to indicate either normal or diseased processes in the body. Body temperature, for example, is a well-known biomarker for fever, and cholesterol level is a biomarker for heart disease. In Alzheimer's disease, several biomarkers have emerged that appear critical to early recognition, including structural changes in the brain (like decreased size of the hippocampus), results of actual imaging of amyloid in the brain, spinal fluid abnormalities, and genetic markers. But in an editorial, Alzheimer's specialists Ronald Petersen, PhD, MD, and John Trojanowski, MD, PhD, argue that while biomarker data will likely be integrated with imaging and clinical data to use for predictive testing for AD, it is premature to get too excited insofar as real patient care is concerned: "Of critical importance, however, is what the clinician and patient will do with the results. Alzheimer disease has no treatment to prevent or alter the course of the disease, so making the diagnosis with good accuracy may aid in planning but could also be devastating news for some patients and families."[11]

An important goal of most memory clinics is to enroll patients in clinical treatment trials. The Alzheimer's Association in particular promotes participation in clinical trials. The following was taken directly from their website and is used by permission.[12]

Reasons to consider participating

You can make a difference! Clinical studies are the engine that powers medical progress. Scientists work constantly to find better ways to treat diseases. Improved treatments can never become a reality without testing in human volunteers. No one ever chooses to become ill, but anyone can consider helping to advance knowledge about an illness affecting them or someone close to them.

There is reason for optimism about experimental treatments. No investigational treatment advances to clinical testing unless there is strong evidence indicating it will be as good or better than currently available therapies.

Every study matters. Every clinical study contributes valuable knowledge, whether or not the treatment works as hoped.

Participants receive a high standard of care. All participants receive regular care related to the study and opportunities to talk to study staff. Research shows that people involved in studies tend to do somewhat better than people in a similar stage of their disease who are not enrolled, regardless of whether the experimental treatment works. Scientists believe this advantage may be due to the general high quality of care provided during clinical studies.

As with most aspects of dementia care, there are both pros and cons to participating in clinical trails, and my goal is to point out some aspects that aren't usually discussed by those hoping to recruit volunteers. Clinical trials are the primary way that researchers find out if a promising treatment is safe and effective for patients. They take place at private research facilities, teaching hospitals, specialized AD research centers, and doctors' offices. An excellent discussion of dementia clinical trials in question and answer format may be found at the National Institutes on Aging website.[13]

Certainly the need for trial participants is staggering. According to the National Institute on Aging, today "at least 50,000 volunteers both with and without Alzheimer's are urgently needed to participate in more than 175 actively enrolling Alzheimer's disease clinical trials and studies in the US. To reach that goal, researchers will have to screen at least half a million potential volunteers."

In my experience, participation in a dementia clinical trial is best viewed by patients and caregivers as a terrific opportunity to contribute to knowledge that will help *future* patients rather then themselves. It is an altruistic endeavor that is essential if meaningful progress is to be made in the field. The other significant benefit is regular contact with the study team. Team members may become an invaluable source of support, advice, and education. In fact, the positive influence of the study team on the person with dementia is often cited as an important reason that patients on *placebo* improve in measurable ways over the course of the study, making it more difficult for the active study medication to show statistical improvement over placebo. In fact, my fondest memories from my involvement as an investigator several years ago in an assisted living trial studying the atypical antipsychotic medication risperidone (Risperdal) versus placebo in the treatment of dementia-related psychosis were the relationships I developed with study participants, their families, and the study coordinator. Recruitment of patients into this study was extremely difficult, with most turning down the opportunity. Most clinical trials today are rigorously designed, and the frequency of required visits, laboratory studies, and rating scale administration may make it difficult for study participants and their families to make it through to the end of the study.

An analogy may be drawn to clinical trials in the cancer field. In a revealing front-page article in the August 3, 2009 edition of the *New York Times*, it is noted that there are more than 6,500 cancer clinical trials seeking adult patients, and that many will be abandoned along the way. In addition, "more than one trial in five sponsored by the National Cancer Institute failed to enroll a single subject." The problem is stated bluntly in the article: "Most patients are not interested in clinical trials. Some do not want the extra office visits and tests a trial entails and do not want their treatment determined by the flip of a coin. Others fear getting a placebo . . . Others find the whole idea too overwhelming when they are trying to save their lives."[14]

Another word of caution applies to the need for the utmost integrity of those involved as study investigators. In part due to the rigorous nature of most clinical trials, compensation for patient recruitment, enrollment, and study completion may be lucrative, and these financial incentives may foster questionable behaviors. For example, some memory clinics may be set up with the sole aim of recruiting patients into clinical trials, although this aim may not be what is advertised. In response to criticism of memory clinics as sites for recruiting subjects for drug trials, a letter published in the *British Medical Journal* in March 2009 fired back the following:

> Critics are right to question the evidence base for memory clinics if the only purpose for memory clinics is to screen for drug treatments. However, they also provide an acceptable, accessible, high quality assessment, rehabilitation, and follow-up facility for people with memory concerns or suspected dementia and their families. If dementia is construed as a common long term disability of later life, then memory clinics can neutralize the double stigma of age and dementia and provide timely interventions that help people and their families to live well with the condition.[15]

Obviously, many people concerned about memory problems don't have easy access to bona fide memory clinics. But this needn't dissuade you from taking some action to determine if a problem really exists that warrants further testing.

We're now ready to review the primary "reality lessons" learned about memory clinics and clinical trials so that you will be able to make a better decision about whether they're right for your particular situation.

LESSON 1: STRENGTHS AND WEAKNESSES OF MEMORY CLINICS

Strategies

1. Realize that memory clinics are generally best used for early assessment and diagnosis, while treatment of behavioral disturbances and psychoses in more advanced dementia patients is not usually a memory clinic strength.
2. Don't be unduly swayed or influenced by access to state-of-the-art imaging and testing technologies. It may be that practical advice, education, and awareness of behavioral strategies may be more relevant and helpful in your situation.
3. Take advantage of the resources available from most memory clinics: information, support, links with other agencies, referrals to other experts, links to religious and spiritual services, local lectures, and so on. Inquire about how off-hours crises are handled and whether 24-hour telephone support is available.

LESSON 2: REALISTIC EXPECTATIONS

Strategies

1. Recognize what the objectives of most memory clinics are: early diagnosis and treatment, identifying other disorders that may be contributing to memory problems, evaluating new therapies via clinical trials, and reassuring the "worried well."
2. Have one or two goals in mind related to what you hope to gain from enrolling in a memory clinic and share these goals with the staff at the initial meeting/assessment period. This will minimize the chances of disappointment and frustration with the memory clinic experience.

LESSON 3: CLINICAL TRIALS

Strategies

1. Be prepared for the clinic to try to recruit your loved one to participate in clinical trials. While trials are essential in moving the field toward finding a cure, they may or may not be right for your individual situation.
2. Ask the tough questions that may not be spelled out: What are my options when the trial ends? What if the drug really helped but it's not yet available on the market? What if side effects or other reasons lead me to want to drop out of the study? and Are my regular doctors restricted from changing my medications while I'm enrolled in the study?

9

MENTAL CAPACITY AND DECISION MAKING IN DEMENTIA: THE CHANGING OF THE WILL

Of all the aspects of dementia care that I have been involved with over the years, none have been more interesting and at times strange than cases involving mental capacity and decision making, with making a will being one of the more important examples of decision-making capacity. After a brief summary of health care proxies and decision-making authority for people with Alzheimer's disease (AD), I will attempt to prepare you for a world that, should you decide to enter it, will likely be more bizarre and unpredictable than you could ever have imagined. I'll share details from several cases that I've been personally involved in as well as relevant points from a prominent recent case that has been featured in the mass media.

Of the many reasons early diagnosis of Alzheimer's disease is important, having time to get your advance directives in order is one of the most important. The term "advance directives" refers to preferences about treatment and the designation of a surrogate decision maker in the event you should become unable to make decisions yourself. One type of advance directive, known as a living will, can specify the types of treatments and procedures that you want or don't want to receive if you should become terminally ill or go into a vegetative state.

One of the most important types of advance directives is the designation of a health care proxy, someone who can make your health care decisions if you become mentally incapacitated. Often referred to as a durable power of attorney (POA) for health care, this legal document designates a person to make health care decisions for you. Unlike a living will, it is not limited to end-of-life situations.

A durable power of attorney becomes effective when it is signed, and it continues indefinitely, although you may revoke it at any time as long as you still have mental capacity. A key reason to act early is that once you lose the mental capacity to understand the nature and consequences of your actions, you are no longer able to execute a valid power of attorney. These situations may require the appointment of a legal guardian or conservator, which may severely restrict your rights.

Mental capacity is a world where the fields of law and medicine intersect, fields that seem to use two different languages. If you think doctors use medical jargon that makes it difficult to understand and retain information, consider the legal jargon found in the world of probate courts and rulings on mental capacity. The following summary taken from *Texas Legal Standards Related to Mental Capacity in Guardianship Proceedings*, should illustrate my point:

> In the seminal case *Missouri Pacific Railroad Co. v. Brazil*, 10 S. W. 403, 406 (Tex. 1888), the Texas Supreme Court examined whether the party had mental capacity sufficient to comprehend the nature, purpose, and effect of the contract and held that if a person lacking mental capacity executes a contract and is subsequently restored to reason and acts as to clearly evidence his intention to be bound by the contract, the law will regard the contract as ratified.[1]

MENTAL CAPACITY

On the face of it, the concept of mental capacity seems reasonably straight-forward: a person either knows what he or she is doing or he or she doesn't. People possess mental capacity in varying degrees. While "mental capacity" eludes precise definition, it includes elements of memory, logic, reason, and calculating. Capacity can and does fluctuate, and it is usually viewed as task specific. So, for example, as noted in the journal article "Ten Myths about Decision-Making Capacity," a patient with mild dementia might be able to decide that she wants antibiotic treatment for a urinary tract infection because the treatment:

> allows her to pursue important goals such as feeling well or staying out of the hospital, and its burdens and risks are low. On the other hand, the same patient might be unable to weigh the multiple risks and benefits of a complex neurosurgical procedure with uncertain tradeoffs between quality and quantity of life. Therefore, when evaluating a patient's capacity to make healthcare decisions, clinicians must assess each decision separately.[2]

In real life, of course, assessing every decision separately is impractical and may even evolve into a theater of the absurd. In one case I was involved in, the daughter (and durable power of attorney for health care) of an elderly woman in a nursing home with moderate stage Alzheimer's disease was trying to dictate the terms of her mother's care to the staff, including issues such as toileting schedule, activities she should participate in, and which fellow residents she should socialize with. A problem was that her mother was still capable of making many decisions for herself, and so the staff found themselves in a frustrating no-win situation: they could satisfy the daughter or the mother, but not both. So they invited me to be the arbiter: which decisions did mom still have the mental capacity to make, and which did she not still have? I soon realized this would be an impossible and futile exercise, as she would typically make dozens of decisions every day. So my proposed solution was to point out (in writing) several general strengths and weaknesses in the patient's cognitive abilities, and to allow her to continue to make as many daily decisions that the staff felt were reasonable and not harmful to her.

Adults are in fact presumed to be of sound mind and capable of managing their own affairs, and the burden of proof rests with the party alleging mental incapacity. Similarly, elderly persons are presumed competent, which is of course as it should be. Capacity is essential to guardianship cases, as well as cases involving fraud, undue influence (see later in this chapter), financial transactions, mental health commitments, and health care decisions. Specific types of capacity include testamentary capacity, capacity to sign contracts, and testimonial capacity. *Testamentary capacity* is the mental competency to execute a will at the time the will was signed and witnessed. To have testamentary capacity, the author of the will (testator) must understand the nature of making a will, have a general idea of what he or she possesses, and know the members of his or her immediate family or other "natural objects of his/her bounty," those individuals preferred to take ownership of their property at death. Inherent in that capacity is the ability to resist the pressures or domination of any person who may try to use undue influence on the distribution of the testator's (will writer's) estate. Undue influence connotes excessive pressure to act in a way that negates the person's free will. Often, the perpetrator will promise to care for the person if funds or material goods are transferred. Unfortunately, the list of perpetrators is long: family members, caregivers, neighbors, friends, con artists, attorneys, and trustees. As with mental capacity in general, in most states, a testator is *presumed competent* to make a will. For the contesting of the will to be successful, a person challenging the will has the legal burden of proving that the testator was incompetent or unduly influenced. Interestingly, a person under legal guardianship *may* competently make a will, although his or her competency at the time the will was written must be proved.

UNDUE INFLUENCE

Of course, the validity of a will becomes an issue only if the will is contested. Fewer than 3 percent of wills are contested, and 15 percent of those that are contested are overturned. Most wills that are contested are contested by family members who feel they have been slighted; they may have been disinherited, there may be a later will that designates different beneficiaries, or another person becomes involved with the testator whose motivations are questioned. The two legal bases for contesting a will are incompetence (lacking testamentary capacity) and undue influence when making the will. Typically a means to financially exploit the victim, undue influence, as mentioned earlier, connotes excessive pressure to act in a way that negates the person's free will. Estimates of the prevalence of elder financial abuse range from 12 percent to as high as 50 percent. Vulnerability increases with recent bereavement, estrangement from children, physical disability, isolation, depression, and cognitive deficits. The worst predators are those who establish long-term controlling relationships with their elderly victims. They instill paranoia and suspicion in the victim to increase the sense of helplessness and dependency. Assets are gained through deceit, intimidation, and psychological abuse. Business professionals may cheat the victim through bogus investments or financial advice. Consequences are too often devastating, including early death.

In a recent case I was involved in, the daughter of an assisted living facility resident with mild dementia contacted me about her mother's testamentary capacity. It turned out that a year earlier, several months after her husband died, she was approached by her husband's former accountant, who began to build on the trust he had earned from her husband. Eventually, he succeeded in convincing her to change her will and name him as the primary beneficiary. He took advantage of her psychological vulnerability (bereavement-related depression), her financial naïveté (her husband had managed all of their finances), and her insidious cognitive decline. Fortunately, her cognitive deficits were relatively mild, and she retained sufficient insight and judgment to appreciate that she had been essentially swindled. I felt she did in fact possess testamentary capacity, which enabled her to rescind her amended will and restore her original will.

LEGAL GUARDIANS AND CONSERVATORS

Two forces have been colliding in the area of legal guardians and conservators, leading to a growing numbers of cases: increasing numbers of people with cognitive deficits and society's shifting the decision-making burden to the individual. Ironically, recent cases have even involved unethical guardians and conservators engaging in fraud, abuses, and civil rights violations. The positions of guardian and conservator were created to fill a void for people unable or unfit to care for themselves. Although guardians were originally established to look after the needs of orphans, the elderly now comprise 37 to 57 percent of public guardianship wards. Public guardianship programs are often understaffed and underfunded, while cases have become increasingly complicated. Recently, I was asked to assess an 83-year-old man who has been widowed for 17 years but still lives in his own home. A proud father of three and veteran of both the navy and the army, R. B. spends his days doing word puzzles, watching television, and reading the newspaper. His grandson sleeps upstairs in his home, and his son visits frequently and assists with groceries, medication management, and doctor visits. His cognitive deficits are relatively mild, as he scored 25/30 on the Mini-Mental Status Examination (MMSE), with excellent language skills but poor short-term memory. As in many similar situations, he overestimates his abilities and exhibits poor insight and impaired judgment. At age 81, he was exploited financially by both his daughter and granddaughter, who were charged with embezzlement. He was not a particularly wealthy man, relying on both his Social Security check and army retirement check to pay his bills. Since he was found two years earlier (at age 81) to have moderate memory deficits that "prevented him from recalling pertinent factors or information necessary for decision making," a local attorney was appointed as his legal guardian. His son became increasingly frustrated by this arrangement, as it was too complicated for him to deal with checks for groceries, arrangements for doctors visits, and visits from home care agencies when there was a third party involved that was officially R. B.'s legal guardian. Neither R. B. nor his son got along with this attorney, and amid allegations of improprieties, he resigned as guardian several months prior to my involvement, with a temporary guardian appointed shortly thereafter. As it seemed apparent to me and others involved that R. B.'s son clearly had his father's best interests at heart, I stated in my report that it is always preferable to have a trusted family member appointed legal guardian unless there are severe extenuating circumstances. As I stepped back later to think about R. B., it dawned on me that in many ways he was doubly victimized: his own daughter and granddaughter exploited him, but then an imperfect legal system intervened to add insult to injury.

Assessing Mental Capacity

What does it mean to be mentally competent? An important concept is that for a particular decision, the person either is or is not competent to make that particular decision. When performing a mental capacity assessment, one of my primary goals is to determine whether an illness or condition impairs the person's ability to make the decision at hand rationally. A person who is incompetent to balance a checkbook may be perfectly competent to change a will or trust. A person with mild Alzheimer's disease who is incompetent today because her urinary tract infection has caused increased confusion may be competent next week to make the same decision. In and of themselves, diagnoses such as Alzheimer's, schizophrenia, and bipolar disorder shouldn't imply incompetence. Finally, the consequences of a person's decision should be factored in to competency determinations: a person wanting to designate a small part of her estate to an individual should require a lower threshold of capacity than if she wanted to completely change the disposition of her estate in a radical fashion.

Elements of decisional ability usually include understanding, appreciating, reasoning, and making a choice. In the elderly with dementia, of course, functional abilities play a critical role: personal hygiene, proper diet, safety awareness, following medication regimens, performing financial activities, and responding to health problems. Reports from social workers, family members, caregivers, departments of elderly affairs, visiting nurses, and occupational and physical therapists become important. Capacity evaluations should be thorough, with attention paid to the presence of others, the time of day, the setting, and the tests performed. One reason there are so many gray areas in mental capacity assessments is that there is a lack of clear criterion or reference standard of incompetence. While having a diagnosis of dementia doesn't imply incompetence, it certainly merits a thorough assessment. As all neuropsychologists are keenly aware, the importance of *executive functions* can't be overstated in mental capacity cases, that is, higher level cognitive functions that orchestrate relatively simple ideas, movements, or actions into complex, goal-directed behavior.

Unfortunately, as we have seen with so many aspects of dementia, the real world finds a way to confound the textbooks and academicians. Consider the personal expose' entitled "A Family's Fight to Save an Elder from Scammers," published in the June 17, 2009 edition of the *Wall Street Journal*. The writer, Karen Blumenthal, describes the frustration of her own family in trying to protect their loved one, an "Ivy-League educated professional" in his mid-seventies, from financial abuse by scammers. Among other things, he had wired several thousand dollars to strangers, believing he was paying taxes on huge lottery winnings. Despite agreeing to appoint his son as power of attorney for finances, he "continued to send money away he couldn't afford to lose, fully expecting to see a huge reward in a matter of days." His family tried everything: "His children and stepchildren counseled him, cajoled him, and took him to task. Experts, lawyers, and his doctor were consulted. Law-enforcement agencies, from the local police to state officials to the Federal Bureau of Investigation, were called." "We never found a law-enforcement agency that cared," the son says. "To me, nobody gave a damn." Finally, after he was "conned into selling his car and wiring $4000 to Costa Rica," a judge granted legal guardianship to two of his children, "taking away his right to manage his own affairs."[3]

For families and loved ones trying to help, as this article illustrates, the obstacles are enormous, with some less obvious than others. Many elders, for example, *appear on the surface to be extremely sharp*, so trying to convince doctors, law enforcement personnel, and judges that a person is mentally incompetent is extremely challenging. Many physicians find it hard to believe that a person could score 30/30 on the MMSE and still be mentally incapacitated, especially when it comes to finances. A recent study found that declining capacity to manage financial affairs in people with mild cognitive impairment (MCI) may predict a subsequent diagnosis of Alzheimer's disease during the next year. The study used a standardized test, the Financial Capacity Instrument, that looks at a broad range of financial skills from simple to complex. Tasks such as checkbook management and bank statement management are measured. One of the study's recommendations was for clinicians to "proactively monitor patients with MCI for declining financial skills and advise patients and families about appropriate interventions."[4]

While an excellent idea in theory, I've never heard of a clinician who has actually done this; most lack the time or skills to do this type of monitoring, and most people with MCI aren't referred to specialists who might actually monitor them proactively.

THE CASE OF BROOKE ASTOR

In my opinion, the Brooke Astor case is the most notorious and publicized story to come along in recent years to illustrate so many of the themes discussed in this chapter: mental capacity in a person with Alzheimer's disease, testamentary capacity, legal guardianship, financial abuse by a family member (her son) and an attorney, family dysfunction, and the unusual situations that occur when similar cases go to court.

To briefly summarize the case, Brooke Astor, the legendary society doyenne and philanthropist who died in 2007 at age 105, was known to have made more than 30 wills in her lifetime. Prosecutors argued that Brooke Astor's son, Anthony D. Marshall, and his codefendant, Francis X. Morrissey Jr., a lawyer who worked on Mrs. Astor's estate, conspired to take advantage of Mrs. Astor's dementia to coerce her into changing her estate plan. The two men faced a total of 22 charges of conspiracy, scheming to defraud, larceny, and forgery, with the prosecution arguing that Mrs. Astor was not legally competent to make decisions, including changing her will and consenting to the sale of a prized painting. One of the critical issues was whether Mrs. Astor possessed testamentary capacity when she signed her 2002 will, which was amended in late 2003 and again in early 2004. Those revisions gave her son more control over her estate and reduced the amount of money she left to the New York libraries, museums, universities, and parks she spent so much of her life supporting. As noted in the *New York Times*, much of the contention centered on when Mrs. Astor became incompetent: some jurors concluded it didn't occur until 2005, while others believed it happened as early as 2002. But as I explained earlier, competency is not something that is simply lost on a specific date and never regained; a person's capabilities may change with time and treatment. As noted in probate attorney Andrew Mayoras' blog shortly after the jury verdict was announced on October 8, 2009: "I must express my surprise at the will-related convictions. People with Alzheimer's have good and bad days, and proving Astor incompetent at the moment of signing, based on the high proof required in a criminal case (beyond a reasonable doubt), was very hard to do."[5]

The family dysfunction that was involved was even more pronounced than is typical in similar cases. In 2007, Anthony Marshall's son Philip enlisted the support of two of his grandmother's friends, Annette de la Renta and David Rockefeller, to petition the court for legal guardianship of Mrs. Astor, alleging that his father (who was her power of attorney) mistreated her. Included in the petition was the following allegation: "Her bedroom is so cold in the winter that my grandmother is forced to sleep in the TV room in torn nightgowns on a filthy couch that smells, probably from dog urine."[6]

The trial lasted 19 weeks, included over 14,000 pages of transcripts, and involved over 70 witnesses. To illustrate the craziness of it all, Benjamin Brafman, a criminal defense lawyer and former prosecutor, was quoted in the *New York Times* as saying, "The question of competence does not necessarily, in my view, require the testimony of every human being who came into contact with Brooke Astor in the latter years of her life."[7] After the October 8, 2009 jury verdict was read finding Mr. Marshall guilty of 14 of the 16 counts against him and Mr. Morrissey guilty of conspiracy and forgery, the jurors "likened the sordid family drama to a Shakespearean tragedy that left them sick to their stomachs."[8]

Mr. Marshall was found guilty of one of two first-degree grand larceny charges, the most serious he faced. Jurors convicted him of giving himself an unauthorized raise of about $1 million for managing his mother's finances. The prosecution had contended that Mrs. Astor's dementia had advanced to the point that she lacked the mental capacity to approve of this raise and other financial decisions that benefited her son. The defense announced their intention to appeal the verdict.

One of the positive outcomes of the media attention given the trial was the increase in public awareness of elder financial abuse. Elder abuse is any illegal or improper use of an elder's funds, property, or assets. Examples include cashing an elderly person's check without authorization or permission, forging an elderly person's signature, misusing or stealing an older person's money or possessions, or coercing or deceiving an elderly person into signing any document.

The Brooke Astor case reinforces what is often the basis for a board exam question for recertification in geriatric psychiatry: In 55 percent of cases, the perpetrator is a family member, friend, neighbor or caregiver. In fewer cases the perpetrator is a financial professional working for the victim or a scam artist previously unknown to the victim. As noted by Sharon Merriman-Nai, comanager of the National Center on Elder Abuse: "If financial abuse can happen to a rich and famous person like Astor, it can happen to anybody. There are many, many people out there being taken advantage of in much smaller ways. It may be smaller dollar amounts than in the Astor case, but it can be just as devastating in their lives. The point [the trial made was] this occurs everywhere."[9]

ELDER LAW ATTORNEYS

With all of the important legal issues involved in Alzheimer's disease, hiring an expert called an elder law attorney may be well worth the expense. Elder law attorneys have specialized knowledge and experience that personal attorneys may not have. While personal referrals from friends and colleagues may be invaluable, two national organizations may help as well. The National Elder Law Foundation (www.nelf.org) provides board certification with similar requirements for elder law attorneys across the country. Attorneys with that certification will have the initials "CELA" after their names. A second national organization, the National Academy of Elder Law Attorneys (www.naela.org), is a professional association of over 4,200 attorneys who assist their clients with guardianship and conservatorship, probate and estate planning, elder abuse issues, and long-term care planning. Other important issues that elder care attorneys may work on include powers of attorney and living wills, mental capacity issues, resident rights in long-term care facilities, and will and trust planning.

Important considerations in choosing an elder care attorney include how long he or she has been practicing, whether elder law is the attorney's specialty, and what his or her experience is with dementia and cognitive impairment.

Let's now review the main lessons presented in this chapter and strategies to help caregivers ensure that issues of mental capacity don't cause unnecessary grief.

LESSON 1: MENTAL CAPACITY IS NOT A STRAIGHTFORWARD CONCEPT

Strategies

1. Don't assume your doctor, lawyer, or financial advisor adequately understands the concept of mental capacity and can effectively apply it to your loved one's situation. By reading this chapter, you now know more about it than many (if not most) health care professionals. Medical schools do not teach future doctors about these issues, nor do residency training programs.
2. Seek a second opinion if you disagree with the findings in your situation or if you believe your loved one's competency evaluation was inadequate or incomplete. Keep in mind that health insurance usually doesn't cover these types of evaluations.

LESSON 2: BECOMING DURABLE POWER OF ATTORNEY DOESN'T ALWAYS SOLVE THE PROBLEM

Strategies

1. As shown in the Brooke Astor case, the case presented in the *Wall Street Journal*, and many others, power of attorney (POA) isn't always sufficient to prevent elder abuse or to meet your loved one's needs. The individual must have both the capacity to appoint an agent and a trusted person to choose. State statutes differ in other limitations that may apply.

2. Powers of attorney don't in fact have much power after all is said and done. They can be revoked, ignored, or changed by the individual if he or she disagrees with the agent's decisions. In addition, actions taken by a power of attorney are increasingly being scrutinized. A May 2011 *Wall Street Journal* story on powers of attorney noted that "banks, for their part, have started rejecting financial maneuvers made under the cloak of a power of attorney, for fear of being parties to fraud." Of course, this caution by banks may be well and good until your loved one with mild dementia and worsening financial capacity is withdrawing money from the bank to buy hundreds of dollars worth of useless or scam-fueled stuff. Democratic U.S. Senator Herb Kohl of Wisconsin has noted that crimes committed by people with powers of attorney "are the worst kinds of crimes, ranging from credit-card fraud and forgery to outright theft."[10] In view of these issues with power of attorney, it may be appropriate to pursue legal guardianship by contacting an attorney with experience in elder care law. The National Academy of Elder Law Attorneys' website may be found at http://www.naela.com

LESSON 3: BE VIGILANT ABOUT ELDER FINANCIAL ABUSE

Strategies

1. In the August 2011 issue of *Money* magazine, a 2010 study was cited that showed one out every five elderly Americans has been sold an inappropriate investment, paid excessive fees for a financial product or service, or been a victim of fraud. Not only do older people tend to have more time on their hands to browse the Internet and attend free meal seminars, they also tend to have more money: after a lifetime of saving, the average household led by those age 75 years or older has a net worth of $638,000.[11] Being vigilant means you may need to pry a little into your parents' financial affairs and be more involved, or even coach them into how to end a conversation.
2. Be particularly wary about "new friends" that are attempting to develop gradual, trusting relationships that have red flags attached to them. While it may be perfectly legitimate and innocent, it may not be, so when money, gifts, or investments become part of the package, show particular scrutiny and even consider enlisting the help of your loved one's primary care physician.

10

THE SHRINKING WORKFORCE: WHY ISN'T THERE AN OLD AGE DOCTOR IN THE HOUSE?

Imagine having a 7-year-old son with a high fever and being unable to locate a pediatrician to see him. There are just too few, you are told, so you need to take him to another type of practitioner. While this scenario sounds far-fetched, it is not so for the analogous situation on the other end of the age spectrum. In fact, the reality is that the ability to take your elderly parent or spouse with dementia to a geriatrician or geriatric psychiatrist is increasingly becoming a rarity. While institutions that train health care workers responded to twentieth-century demographics and embraced the need to prepare workers in pediatrics, a similar commitment to geriatrics has not occurred. Of the 650,000 licensed physicians practicing in the United States, fewer than 9,000 have met qualifying criteria in geriatrics, a ratio of 2.5 geriatricians to every 10,000 older adults. This compares with approximately 1 pediatrician for every 1,000 children.

For me, choosing a career in geriatric psychiatry was relatively easy; once I decided I would be a psychiatrist, there was no doubt I most wanted to work with the elderly population. For one thing, older people are generally wise, resilient, and lacking in fear of death. They have tremendous life experience, overcoming obstacles many younger people would find insurmountable. As Plato said: "It gives me great pleasure to converse with the aged, they have been over the road that all of us must travel and know where it is rough and difficult and where it is easy and level."

In my view, effective interventions for the elderly are practical and in the here-and-now: medications; short-term psychotherapies such as cognitive-behavioral (CBT), interpersonal (IPT), and problem-solving; and electroconvulsive therapy (ECT). Since the elderly often have multiple medical problems and are often on multiple medications, and since dementia is a disease that often affects people without prior psychiatric problems, I saw it as an opportunity to help destigmatize the field and solidify my identity as a physician rather than a "shrink." Unfortunately, my attraction to the field has not been shared by many others who enter psychiatry.

A fascinating and timely report entitled *Retooling for an Aging America: Building the Health Care Workforce* was released by the prestigious Institute of Medicine in 2008.[1] The Institute of Medicine (IOM) formed the Committee on the Future Health Care Workforce for Older Americans in January 2007 to determine the best use of the health care workforce to meet the needs of the growing number of adults age 65 years or older. To address this charge, the committee sought to describe promising models of health care delivery and the workforce that will be necessary in the future to serve the health care needs of the population of older adults, recognizing that any or all of these needs may change over time. Issues addressed relate both directly and indirectly to those affected by dementia. First of all, increased longevity means more people will develop dementia, since age is far and away the most important risk factor for developing Alzheimer's disease (AD). Second, the report emphasized the heterogeneity of the elderly, with increasing numbers of gay, lesbian, and bisexual elders. The field of geriatrics has not even begun to address those issues of elder heterogeneity in dementia care, which will have increasing relevance in long-term care communities. That current dementia care is suboptimal was also addressed: models shown to be effective and efficient are not widely implemented and payment from any source is lacking for patient education, coordination of care, and geriatric expertise.

The focus of the report was clearly on the workforce issues facing care of the elderly. The statistics presented are startling: there are currently 7,100 geriatricians (a number that declines annually) and 1,600 geriatric psychiatrists. Fewer than 1 percent of nurses and pharmacists specialize in geriatrics, as do less than 4 percent of social workers (see also Chapter 2 for a detailed discussion of nursing home social workers). Consider the route that graduating medical residents take to become geriatricians: they enter a one- or two-year geriatric medicine fellowship. In 2009 273 of the 489 available first-year positions were filled, compared with 290 of 400 available positions in 2003. The comparable statistics for my chosen field, geriatric psychiatry, are even worse: 54 of 120 available first-year fellowship positions were filled in 2009, compared with 95 of 110 available positions in 2000. Explanations provided for these ominous trends include negative stereotypes of older adults, lower incomes for geriatric specialists, and the high cost of training (geriatricians train at least one year longer than their primary care colleagues, and yet they are compensated at a lower level). The median salary for a geriatrician in private practice in 2010 was $183,523. This was $5,879 less than the average family physician's salary, and $21,856 less than the average general internist's. The workers who provide direct care to our elders are inadequately compensated; nationally, personal and home care aides earn an average of $8.54 per hour. These direct care workers have such high turnover rates that overall costs to employers run over $4 billion annually. If I made the case in Chapter 4 that nursing home social workers are not generally well trained, the data for direct care workers are even worse: federal training minimums have not changed in 20 years and "may be lower than for dog groomers, cosmetologists, and crossing guards." Less than 1 percent of registered nurses (RNs) are certified in geriatrics, and only 29 percent of RN baccalaureate programs have a certified faculty member. About 2.6 percent of advanced practice registered nurses (APRNs) are certified in geriatrics, with 300 geriatric APRNs graduating annually. In my organization, we have hired and trained family practice–trained APRNs and physician assistants (PAs) to provide behavioral health services to long-term care facility residents, reflecting both the demand for these services as well as the obvious shortage of geriatric certified providers. Using PAs as an example of a prudent means to meet the demand for our services, The IOM *Aging Report* seems to agree with our strategy. As they note (p. 146), "Physician assistants (PAs) represent an important part of the work-force for the elderly population (Olshansky et al., 2005). PAs work under the supervision of a physician, but they can often work apart from the physician's direct presence and can prescribe medications and bill for health care services. Unlike some of the other professions described above, the PA workforce tends to be younger and is growing rapidly. About half of PAs work in family medicine or general medicine (Brugna et al., 2007; Hooker and Berlin, 2002). The 65-and-older population accounts for about 32 percent of office visits to PAs (Hachmuth and Hootman, 2001), and 78 percent of PAs report treating at least some patients over the age of 85 (Center for Health Workforce Studies, 2005). PAs are an especially important source of care in underserved areas, where they often act as the principal care provider in clinics, with physicians attending on an intermittent basis. In this vein, they are a potential source of care to meet the increased need that is projected for long-term care settings. Their use may be a particularly attractive strategy since, as with NPs, the use of PAs has been shown to be cost-effective (Ackermann and Kemle, 1998; Brugna et al., 2007)." In my experience, PAs are well suited to long-term care work, work that usually requires long hours, broad-based medical knowledge, and strong interpersonal skills. Often PAs are true apprentices, learning the art and skill of long-term care psychiatry through experience, collaboration, and supervision.

Similarly, advanced practice nurses (APRNs) have also been crucial players as we work to treat long-term care residents with dementias and related disorders. An RN may become an APRN by obtaining a master's degree and may become certified either through a national certifying examination or through state certification mechanisms. An APRN functions as an independent health care provider, addressing the full range of a patient's health problems and needs within an area of specialization. There are different types of APRNs, including NPs, who provide primary care; clinical nurse specialists, who typically specialize in a medical or surgical specialty; certified nurse anesthetists; and certified nurse midwives. The pipeline for producing APRNs with a specialization in geriatrics is inadequate to meet the need. As noted in the IOM report, "NPs represent a particularly important component of the workforce caring for older adults because of their ability to provide primary care as well as care for patients prior to, during, and following an acute care hospitalization and also to care for residents in institutional long-term care settings. NPs treat a disproportionate number of older adults—23 percent of office visits and 47 percent of hospital outpatient visits with NPs are made by people 65 and older (Center for Health Workforce Studies, 2005). Furthermore, NPs care for a higher proportion of elderly poor adults than do physicians or physician assistants (Cipher et al., 2006). Finally, NPs have been shown to provide high-quality care and be cost effective" (Hooker et al., 2005; Melin and Bygren, 1992; Mezey et al., 2005). Many of the APNs I have worked with have been terrific: knowledgeable, empathetic, collaborative. Because they are nurses, they are often better able to relate to and educate the nursing staff in the long-term care facilities.

As for physicians, I'm afraid we may be fighting a losing battle. Consider my chosen field, geriatric psychiatry. The American Board of Psychiatry and Neurology (ABPN) recognized geriatric psychiatry as a subspecialty in 1989 and first awarded 10-year certificates of added qualifications in 1991 (ABPN, 2007). In 1996, the ABPN phased out the practice- pathway option (allowing certification without fellowship training) and subsequently reduced postgraduate training requirements from two years to one year. Only 13 percent of all geriatric psychiatrists ever certified became certified after the practice pathway was phased out.

As the geriatric certifications expire, many physicians do not pursue recertification; most of these physicians were certified via the practice pathway. Reasons for not recertifying include retirement, the burden of the process, the cost, and the lack of perceived benefit. In fact, the requirements for recertification are becoming more onerous. Only about half of all physicians certified in geriatric medicine or geriatric psychiatry before 1994 have been recertified (ADGAP, 2005). By comparison, 89 percent of physicians who received specialty certificates in other disciplines from the American Board of Internal Medicine (ABIM) between 1990 and 1995 enrolled in the maintenance of certification process; of those, 81 percent completed the process (ABIM, 2005). The comparable rate of recertification in geriatrics among other health-related professions is unknown.

A consequence of this lack of geriatric expertise in health care is the perpetuation of stereotypes and misinformation about aging and dementia. Ageist attitudes are rampant in our culture, beginning with prominent physicians in the first decade of the twentieth century speaking of aging as an "incurable disease." Dr. Robert Butler, who coined the term "ageism" 35 years ago, wrote in 2004 that "Daily we are witness to, or even unwitting participants in, cruel imagery, jokes, language, and attitudes directed at older people."[2]

I still hear professionals today who believe depression and Alzheimer's disease are a normal part of aging, or who don't take expressions of suicidal thinking in elderly patients seriously.

Fortunately, there are some hopeful developments. A relatively new journal, *Dementia: The International Journal of Social Research and Practice*, began publishing in 2002. One of its goals is to "assist in breaking down the stereotypes and stigma that surrounds a diagnosis of dementia, and its aftermath." Published articles throughout its 10-year existence have included:

"Essay on a Word: A Lived Experience of Dementia" (Sterin, 2002)

"Personal Spirituality of Persons with Early-Stage Dementia"(Katsuno, 2003)

"Make It Easy on Yourself! Advice to Researchers from Someone with Dementia on Being Interviewed" (McKillop & Wilkinson, 2004)

"Expectations and Experience of Moving to a Care Home: Perceptions of Older People with Dementia" (Thein, D'Souza & Sheehan, 2011)

"Stand up for Dementia: Performance, Improvisation and Stand up Comedy as Therapy for People with Dementia; a Qualitative Study" (Stevens, 2012)

Recognizing the scarcity of geriatric leaders, several institutions have developed innovative approaches to spread knowledge of geriatric principles. For example:

- Through a geriatrics training grant in July 2003, Indiana University, the second largest medical school in the country, established the Geriatrics Education Network of Indiana. Aimed at strengthening the geriatric training of 840 medical students, 450 residents, and 223 practicing physicians, it achieved this goal through a train-the-trainer strategy.
- In 1997, the Practicing Physician Education Project used geriatric experts to train nongeriatrician physician leaders to educate their peers on various geriatric syndromes.
- Since 1992, the Nurses Improving Care for Health System Elders (NICHE) program has worked with nurses in hospital settings to implement models and protocols that improve the care of geriatric patients. In the Geriatric Resource Nurse (GRN) model, a geriatric APN trains a staff nurse to be the clinical resource on geriatric issues for other nurses.

Let's now summarize the key themes presented in this chapter and the strategies caregivers can use to best respond to the troubling workforce trends in dementia care.

LESSON 1: YOU NEEDN'T DESPAIR ABOUT THE SHORTAGE OF GERIATRIC-TRAINED PHYSICIANS

Strategies

1. Think carefully about your unique situation and what you're hoping to accomplish for your loved one: diagnosis, treatment of behavior problems, home health assistance, overall medical care, dementia medications. The more

specifically you can narrow your focus, the better you'll be able to identify resources in your community that may help.

2. It's not about the degree: in dementia care, practitioners such as APNs and PAs who have experience and a collaborative practice environment may be more helpful than a physician who lacks such experience.

LESSON 2: REALIZE THAT DEMENTIA CARE REALLY IS DIFFERENT

Strategies

1. Having dementia really isn't just having "another diagnosis," adding one to a list that may include hypertension, arthritis, chronic obstructive pulmonary disease (COPD), or coronary artery disease. For professionals to manage dementia care well, they must truly possess more than textbook knowledge: experience, empathy, interpersonal skills, interviewing skills, and open-mindedness are all traits to look for when seeking help.

2. Doctors age too, and the fact that someone's been your loved one's doctor for 30 years doesn't imply he or she knows how to handle Alzheimer's disease. Don't passively accept substandard care because it's the path of least resistance and you don't want to offend someone. The era of "the doctor knows best" is gone.

LESSON 3: CHOOSE THE RIGHT PROFESSIONAL TO MEET YOUR NEEDS

Strategies

1. When it comes to dementia care, it doesn't take long to realize how fragmented and chaotic the system is. To negotiate it properly requires knowledge and tenacity. A primary care physician is often the best place to start, but be aware that he or she may downplay or minimize your concerns.

2. Depending on the availability of the following specialists in your area, you should use this as a basic guide to help determine whose strengths are best suited to your individual circumstances.

   a. *Geriatric psychiatrist*: a physician specializing in the mental, emotional, and behavioral disorders affecting the elderly; prescribes medications, treats dementia routinely, and typically completes a residency program in general adult psychiatry; may have completed a fellowship program in geriatric psychiatry

   b. *Geriatrician:* a physician specializing in the health care needs and diseases common among older adults; may serve as primary care physician for older patients or provide specialty consultations; typically completes a residency program in internal medicine followed by a fellowship in geriatric medicine

   c. *Neurologist:* a physician specializing in diseases of the nervous system, including epilepsy, Parkinson's disease, strokes, neuromuscular diseases, and dementias; completes a residency program in neurology; may or may not have specific expertise in older adults and management of dementia-related behavioral problems

d. *Geropsychologist:* a psychologist specializing in the psychological, biological, and social aspects of aging; may provide cognitive therapy, behavioral management strategies, and other therapies related to aging, such as grief and bereavement; doesn't prescribe medications but has a doctorate in psychology and extensive internship experience of supervised practice with older adults

e. *Neuropsychologist:* a psychologist specializing in the relationships between the brain and behavior; typically focuses on the use of psychological tests and assessment techniques to diagnose specific cognitive and behavioral disorders; doesn't prescribe medications but has a doctorate in psychology and extensive internship experience in neuropsychology; may or may not have specific experience and training in disorders affecting the elderly such as dementia

f. *Gerontologist:* a professional specializing in the biological, psychological, and social aspects of aging; typically has a master's degree in gerontology and provides nonmedical services to older adults, such as caregiver education and support groups for both caregivers and people diagnosed with Alzheimer's disease; not medical professionals but do provide important support services that supplement medical care

g. *Advanced practice nurse:* a nurse with advanced didactic and clinical education, knowledge, skills, and scope of practice; roles are regulated by legislation and specific professional regulations that allow for prescribing of medications; those that treat dementia typically are either nurse practitioners or clinical nurse specialists; gerontologic nurse practitioners specialize in the care of older adults

11

REASONS FOR HOPE: STRATEGIES FOR IMPROVING QUALITY OF LIFE FOR THOSE AFFECTED BY DEMENTIA

As with many aspects of dementia, the concept of quality of life has been explored in the academic literature. A 2003 review article cited 14 articles from 1966 to 2002 that identified and reviewed nine different dementia quality of life (QOL) scales.[1] The Cornell-Brown Scale for Quality of Life in Dementia, for example, was developed based on the idea that high QOL is indicated by the presence of positive affect, physical and psychological satisfactions, self-esteem, and the relative absence of negative affect and experiences. The Quality of Life-Alzheimer's Disease scale is composed of 13 items that measure the domains of physical condition, mood, memory, functional abilities, interpersonal relationships, ability to participate in meaningful activities, financial situation, and global assessments of self as a whole and QOL as a whole. These items seem to capture most of what I would deem to be important contributors to quality of life in dementia. My intention here in the final chapter is not to examine these and other scales and debate the merits and scientific validity of each. Rather, I hope to provide useful and practical concepts and strategies to improve the well-being of the person with dementia. In turn, these strategies will likely improve the quality of life of the caregiver as well. I will also show that despite the many challenges, there are reasons for hope that for people with dementia and their families, progress truly is being made in many aspects of dementia care.

Before turning to the actual strategies, let's take a closer look at the caregiver. The following is an excerpt from "Please Don't Ever Put Me in a Nursing Home!" by Debra Stang:

> The woman in the admissions office of the nursing home was white and shaking as she mechanically signed the papers to admit her mother to our facility.

"I promised her," she whispered, reaching for a tissue. "I promised her I would never, ever do this to her."

Meanwhile, as the daughter sat sobbing in the office, her mother, who suffered from dementia, had already been coaxed into a spirited game of Bingo and was having a fine time. During the two years she lived in the facility, she made friends, participated in every kind of activity imaginable, and never uttered one word of complaint about being in a nursing home. In fact, she referred to her new home as "the resort."

But her daughter was never able to let go of the guilt of breaking her promise to her mother. Even after her mother had peacefully passed away in her sleep, the daughter continued to torture herself daily with the broken promise. She died less than six months after her mother.[2]

As I explored in detail in Chapter 3, caregiver stress and burden in dementia are so common that I suspect it is rare for them to be absent. Obvious signs and symptoms include denial about the illness, anger at the person with dementia, social withdrawal, anxiety, depression, exhaustion, somatic complaints, and other health problems. Remarkably, as I mentioned in Chapter 3, a recent study found that the caregiving spouse had *a six-fold increase in dementia risk* compared with subjects whose spouses did not have dementia. This risk was identical for men and women, and it remained after the effects of other dementia risk factors was removed.[3]

I hope this book most helps you with becoming an educated and informed caregiver. To help further that education, I'd like to conclude with ten strategies and suggestions that I hope may prove useful and practical in negotiating the trials and tribulations of dementia.

1. *Become a helpful and integral part of the caregiving team.* Hospitals are building on a movement known as family-centered care, where families are viewed not as visitors, but as a key part of the medical team. A feature story in the October 27, 2009 edition of the *Wall Street Journal* describes this model as it exists in the neonatal intensive care unit (NICU) at St. Louis Children's Hospital. Asking families "Where did you get the baby's middle name," "immediately establishes that the family has information the doctor doesn't know, and it doesn't require a lot of medical terminology."[4] Apply this principle to your chosen nursing home: share your loved one's accomplishments, hobbies, interests, and personality quirks with the staff. Attend as many of the care plan meetings as possible, coming prepared with both realistic concerns and suggestions for improvement.

2. *Encourage supportive management and recognition of staff.* There have been some encouraging recent efforts to decrease staff turnover and foster job satisfaction. At the Emerald Coast Center, a 115-bed skilled nursing facility in Ft. Walton Beach, Florida, seven of the 103 employees have been with the facility for more than 25 years, and another 24 have been on staff for at least 10 years. According to the facility's administrator, Melissa Fijalkowski, staff respond to gestures of gratitude. She periodically mails notes of gratitude to the homes of staff members as a way to express appreciation for a job well done. After

30 days on the job, new hires are asked if the facility is living up to their expectations and what things are going well. Another skilled nursing facility in Denver hires a massage therapist for two hours each week to "give rubdowns to facility staff on the house."[5] As family members, it is important to acknowledge the difficult and stressful nature of the work, take a collaborative as opposed to an adversarial approach, and do whatever you can to facilitate more staff training and education.

3. *Don't underestimate the importance of transitions.* Just as it may take four to six weeks for residents to adjust to a new environment, it may take just as long for the staff to get to know the residents and feel comfortable caring for them. Often during these transitions, families may "test" the staff with demands or requests that appear unreasonable. What is likely occurring is the family is working to trust the staff so that they may have some peace of mind that they have left their loved one in good hands. Often a transition that seems destined for failure actually evolves into a comfortable relationship that inevitably bodes well for the resident's well-being.

4. *Adapt to certain realities of nursing home life.* Most nursing home residents really do have dementia. They may become agitated or aggressive, and they likely have daily fluctuations in lucidity. Overall, nursing home residents are more medically compromised and generally more medically complicated than they were 10 years ago. However, many aspects of nursing home care are improving. Citing data from the Office of the Inspector General, the 2009 Annual Quality Report released by the American Health Care Association (AHCA) and the Alliance for Quality Nursing Home Care found many improvements in quality indicators since 1999. For example, the percentage of residents losing weight dropped 19.55 percent to 9.9 percent, the prevalence of dehydration dropped 81.3 percent to 0.3 percent, and the prevalence of little to no activity dropped 76 percent.

5. *Don't view all psychiatric medications as evil.* While it is true that the interventions for dementia-related behavioral disturbances that carry the least risk are non-pharmacologic ones, they are *sometimes even more effective* when combined with appropriate medications. Similarly, the current approaches to pharmacologic treatment of dementias really have been shown to modestly improve aspects of cognition, function and behavior, and generally the earlier treatment is begun the better the chances of achieving benefits. The tide may even be beginning to turn for the atypical antipsychotic medications often used to treat dementia-related psychosis and behavioral problems. Consider another paper presented at the July 2009 International Alzheimer's Disease Conference in Vienna, Austria, *The Association of Antipsychotic Drug Use and Mortality in the Very Old with Dementia, the Monzino 80+ Study.* This paper reported on an ongoing study of all people age 80 years or older in a province in Italy where 618 participants with dementia (19%) used antipsychotic medications. After four years, the death rate in the antipsychotic use population was 64 percent, compared with 67 percent in the group that didn't use antipsychotics. So it appeared that there was no higher mortality rate in the antipsychotic use group, a promising (albeit preliminary) finding that contradicts results of earlier studies.[6]

6. *Learn as many of the important things as you can about the facility.* Don't be distracted by the aesthetics; rather, focus on the meaningful aspects of dementia care: caring, qualified, and educated staff; good communication with and access to quality health care providers; varied and plentiful activities and programs; and supportive management that truly strives for staff satisfaction and low turnover. Programs that include exercise, music, reminiscing, pet therapy, and others are promising. Even though it may be rare to find a facility with all of these strengths, at least you can make an informed decision and not just go to the one that's the shortest drive from your house.

7. Be aware that in addition to drug development, many exciting and promising *innovations are occurring* in other aspects of dementia care.

   A terrific article in the November 19, 2009 Personal Journal Section of the *Wall Street Journal* entitled "A Key for Unlocking Memories" explored the benefits of music therapy for people with Alzheimer's disease. While noting that "caregivers have observed for decades that Alzheimer's patients can still remember and sing songs long after they've stopped recognizing names and faces," author Melinda Beck points to growing evidence that listening to music can also help stimulate seemingly lost memories and even help restore some cognitive function.[7]

   Similarly, in an effort to incorporate promising developments in the field of neurocognitive rehabilitation, psychologists are developing specific cognitive therapies aimed at patients with dementia. These strategies, including cognitive remediation and cognitive adaptation, are often integrated with physical, occupational, and speech therapies to enhance outcomes in cognitive functioning as well as these other rehabilitation modalities.

   Consider the progress being made in other countries and realize that you can learn from what others are doing. South Korea, as mentioned in Chapter 8, is making great strides in recognizing the disease early, educating its population, and destigmatizing Alzheimer's disease. South Korea's "war on dementia" involves not only education and emphasizing early recognition, but also real hands-on experience.

8. *Act to change the fact that almost half of all emergency department visits and hospital admissions from nursing homes are inappropriate.* One reason for this is the simple fact that facilities often do not communicate with the resident's family, primary care physician, or behavioral health provider. You can prevent this from happening by planning in advance for a situation that may lead to hospitalization. While psychiatric inpatient units certainly have a role in the treatment of dementia-related behavior problems, they may also be overused and even detrimental to the resident's overall quality of life. You can seek out the long-term care facilities that actually have trained clinicians available to intervene in a timely and appropriate manner.

9. *Realize that complacency often leads to mediocrity.* Many examples of this occur in dementia care, especially as a result of dementia's progressive nature, making it a disease that changes with time, environment, and other factors. A medication for aggression and agitation that worked a year ago may no longer be effective; a medication for depression or anxiety that helped six months ago may now require a higher dose. Your loved one with dementia may have derided bingo or pet therapy in the past, but these activities may now be

contributing to positive quality of life. To advocate for your loved one means that from time to time you need to challenge the status quo and encourage others to do the same.

10. *If there is a villain here, my wish is that it be the disease rather than the system and its components.* If I've succeeded in meeting my goals for this book, you are now in a much better position to understand and negotiate the various systems of dementia care that exist. Despite the challenges of the various institutions and individuals that you and your loved one may interact with, you are now able to concentrate on the real issues to ensure the high quality of life that you and your loved one deserve.

APPENDIX: SELECT SECTIONS OF CURRENT NURSING HOME FEDERAL REGULATIONS

Nursing homes that participate in the Medicare and Medicaid programs are subject to federal regulations regarding residents and staff. A report issued in September 2008 found that over 90 percent of nursing homes were cited for federal health or safety violations in 2007, with about 17 percent of nursing homes having deficiencies causing "actual harm or immediate jeopardy" to residents. Complaints about conditions in nursing homes to inspectors number in the tens of thousands every year, and in 2007, 39 percent of the complaints were substantiated.[1]

Nursing homes rank right up there with aviation and nuclear power plants as one of the most highly regulated industries in the United States. So it should come as no surprise that just getting through the regulations faced by nursing homes is daunting. I must admit that because so much time and effort go into complying with these regulations, it sometimes seems that actually improving individual residents' quality of life gets lost in the regulatory morass. To help in sorting through the voluminous nursing home regulations in effect, I've decided to list select sections of current federal regulations for nursing homes that are most relevant for residents with dementia and their caregivers.

The Code of Federal Regulations (CFR) presents the official and complete text of agency regulations in an organized fashion in one publication. It is published by the Office of the Federal Register, an agency of the National Archives and Records Administration. The CFR is divided into 50 titles covering broad subject areas of federal regulations, and nursing home regulations are found in Title 42: Public Health, in Chapter IV: Centers for Medicare and Medicaid Services, Department of Health and Human Services. Part 483 is entitled Requirements for States and Long Term Care Facilities, and the five most relevant sections are presented here, including resident rights, admission, transfer and discharge rights, resident behavior and facility practices, quality of life, and quality of care. The requirements may be found in their entirety here: http://www.access.gpo.gov/nara/cfr/waisidx_02/42cfr483_02.html.

Sec. 483.10 Resident rights.

The resident has a right to a dignified existence, self-determination, and communication with and access to persons and services inside and outside the facility. A facility must protect and promote the rights of each resident, including each of the following rights:

a) Exercise of rights.
    1) The resident has the right to exercise his or her rights as a resident of the facility and as a citizen or resident of the United States.
    2) The resident has the right to be free of interference, coercion, discrimination, and reprisal from the facility in exercising his or her rights.
    3) In the case of a resident adjudged incompetent under the laws of a State by a court of competent jurisdiction, the rights of the resident are exercised by the person appointed under State law to act on the resident's behalf.
    4) In the case of a resident who has not been adjudged incompetent by the State court, any legal-surrogate designated in accordance with State law may exercise the resident's rights to the extent provided by State law.
b) Notice of rights and services.
    1) The facility must inform the resident both orally and in writing in a language that the resident understands of his or her rights and all rules and regulations governing resident conduct and responsibilities during the stay in the facility. The facility must also provide the resident with the notice (if any) of the State developed under section 1919(e)(6) of the Act. Such notification must be made prior to or upon admission and during the resident's stay. Receipt of such information, and any amendments to it, must be acknowledged in writing;
    2) The resident or his or her legal representative has the right—
        i) Upon an oral or written request, to access all records pertaining to himself or herself including current clinical records within 24 hours (excluding weekends and holidays); and
        ii) After receipt of his or her records for inspection, to purchase at a cost not to exceed the community standard photocopies of the records or any portions of them upon request and 2 working days advance notice to the facility.
    3) The resident has the right to be fully informed in language that he or she can understand of his or her total health status, including but not limited to, his or her medical condition;
    4) The resident has the right to refuse treatment, to refuse to participate in experimental research, and to formulate an advance directive as specified in paragraph (8) of this section; and
    5) The facility must—
        i) Inform each resident who is entitled to Medicaid benefits, in writing, at the time of admission to the nursing facility or, when the resident becomes eligible for Medicaid of—

A) The items and services that are included in nursing facility services under the State plan and for which the resident may not be charged;

B) Those other items and services that the facility offers and for which the resident may be charged, and the amount of charges for those services; and

ii) Inform each resident when changes are made to the items and services specified in paragraphs (5)(i) (A) and (B) of this section.

6) The facility must inform each resident before, or at the time of admission, and periodically during the resident's stay, of services available in the facility and of charges for those services, including any charges for services not covered under Medicare or by the facility's per diem rate.

7) The facility must furnish a written description of legal rights which includes—

i) A description of the manner of protecting personal funds, under paragraph (c) of this section;

ii) A description of the requirements and procedures for establishing eligibility for Medicaid, including the right to request an assessment under section 1924(c) which determines the extent of a couple's non-exempt resources at the time of institutionalization and attributes to the community spouse an equitable share of resources which cannot be considered available for payment toward the cost of the institutionalized spouse's medical care in his or her process of spending down to Medicaid eligibility levels;

iii) A posting of names, addresses, and telephone numbers of all pertinent State client advocacy groups such as the State survey and certification agency, the State licensure office, the State ombudsman program, the protection and advocacy network, and the Medicaid fraud control unit; and (iv) A statement that the resident may file a complaint with the State survey and certification agency concerning resident abuse, neglect, misappropriation of resident property in the facility, and non-compliance with the advance directives requirements.

8) The facility must comply with the requirements specified in subpart I of part 489 of this chapter relating to maintaining written policies and procedures regarding advance directives. These requirements include provisions to inform and provide written information to all adult residents concerning the right to accept or refuse medical or surgical treatment and, at the individual's option, formulate an advance directive. This includes a written description of the facility's policies to implement advance directives and applicable State law. Facilities are permitted to contract with other entities to furnish this information but are still legally responsible for ensuring that the requirements of this section are met. If an adult individual is incapacitated at the time of admission and is unable to receive information (due to the incapacitating condition or a mental disorder) or articulate whether or not he or she has executed an advance directive, the facility may give advance

directive information to the individual's family or surrogate in the same manner that it issues other materials about policies and procedures to the family of the incapacitated individual or to a surrogate or other concerned persons in accordance with State law. The facility is not relieved of its obligation to provide this information to the individual once he or she is no longer incapacitated or unable to receive such information. Follow-up procedures must be in place to provide the information to the individual directly at the appropriate time.

9)   The facility must inform each resident of the name, specialty, and way of contacting the physician responsible for his or her care.

10)   The facility must prominently display in the facility written information, and provide to residents and applicants for admission oral and written information about how to apply for and use Medicare and Medicaid benefits, and how to receive refunds for previous payments covered by such benefits.

11)   Notification of changes.

   i)   A facility must immediately inform the resident; consult with the resident's physician; and if known, notify the resident's legal respresentative or an interested family member when there is—

      A)   An accident involving the resident which results in injury and has the potential for requiring physician intervention;

      B)   A significant change in the resident's physical, mental, or psychosocial status (i.e., a deterioration in health, mental, or psychosocial status in either life-threatening conditions or clinical complications);

      C)   A need to alter treatment significantly (i.e., a need to discontinue an existing form of treatment due to adverse consequences, or to commence a new form of treatment); or

      D)   A decision to transfer or discharge the resident from the facility as specified in Sec. 483.12(a).

   ii)   The facility must also promptly notify the resident and, if known, the resident's legal representative or interested family member when there is—

      A)   A change in room or roommate assignment as specified in Sec. 483.15(e)(2); or

      B)   A change in resident rights under Federal or State law or regulations as specified in paragraph (b)(1) of this section.

   iii)   The facility must record and periodically update the address and phone number of the resident's legal representative or interested family member.

c)   Protection of resident funds.

1)   The resident has the right to manage his or her financial affairs, and the facility may not require residents to deposit their personal funds with the facility.

2)   Management of personal funds. Upon written authorization of a resident, the facility must hold, safeguard, manage, and account for the

personal funds of the resident deposited with the facility, as specified in paragraphs (c)(3)-(8) of this section.

3) Deposit of funds.

i) Funds in excess of $50. The facility must deposit any residents' personal funds in excess of $50 in an interest bearing account (or accounts) that is separate from any of the facility's operating accounts, and that credits all interest earned on resident's funds to that account. (In pooled accounts, there must be a separate accounting for each resident's share.)

ii) Funds less than $50. The facility must maintain a resident's personal funds that do not exceed $50 in a non-interest bearing account, interest-bearing account, or petty cash fund.

4) Accounting and records. The facility must establish and maintain a system that assures a full and complete and separate accounting, according to generally accepted accounting principles, of each resident's personal funds entrusted to the facility on the resident's behalf.

i) The system must preclude any commingling of resident funds with facility funds or with the funds of any person other than another resident.

ii) The individual financial record must be available through quarterly statements and on request to the resident or his or her legal representative.

5) Notice of certain balances. The facility must notify each resident that receives Medicaid benefits—

i) When the amount in the resident's account reaches $200 less than the SSI resource limit for one person, specified in section 1611(a)(3)(B) of the Act; and

ii) That, if the amount in the account, in addition to the value of the resident's other nonexempt resources, reaches the SSI resource limit for one person, the resident may lose eligibility for Medicaid or SSI.

6) Conveyance upon death. Upon the death of a resident with a personal fund deposited with the facility, the facility must convey within 30 days the resident's funds, and a final accounting of those funds, to the individual or probate jurisdiction administering the resident's estate.

7) Assurance of financial security. The facility must purchase a surety bond, or otherwise provide assurance satisfactory to the Secretary, to assure the security of all personal funds of residents deposited with the facility.

8) Limitation on charges to personal funds. The facility may not impose a charge against the personal funds of a resident for any item or service for which payment is made under Medicaid or Medicare (except for applicable deductible and coinsurance amounts). The facility may charge the resident for requested services that are more expensive than or in excess of covered services in accordance with Sec. 489.32 of this chapter. (This does not affect the prohibition on facility charges for items and services for which Medicaid has paid. See Sec. 447.15, which limits participation in the Medicaid program to providers who accept,

as payment in full, Medicaid payment plus any deductible, coinsurance, or copayment required by the plan to be paid by the individual.)

i) Services included in Medicare or Medicaid payment. During the course of a covered Medicare or Medicaid stay, facilities may not charge a resident for the following categories of items and services:

A) Nursing services as required at Sec. 483.30 of this subpart.

B) Dietary services as required at Sec. 483.35 of this subpart.

C) An activities program as required at Sec. 483.15(f) of this subpart.

D) Room/bed maintenance services.

E) Routine personal hygiene items and services as required to meet the needs of residents, including, but not limited to, hair hygiene supplies, comb, brush, bath soap, disinfecting soaps or specialized cleansing agents when indicated to treat special skin problems or to fight infection, razor, shaving cream, toothbrush, toothpaste, denture adhesive, denture cleaner, dental floss, moisturizing lotion, tissues, cotton balls, cotton swabs, deodorant, incontinence care and supplies, sanitary napkins and related supplies, towels, washcloths, hospital gowns, over the counter drugs, hair and nail hygiene services, bathing, and basic personal laundry.

F) Medically-related social services as required at Sec. 483.15 (g) of this subpart.

ii) Items and services that may be charged to residents' funds. Listed below are general categories and examples of items and services that the facility may charge to residents' funds if they are requested by a resident, if the facility informs the resident that there will be a charge, and if payment is not made by Medicare or Medicaid:

A) Telephone.

B) Television/radio for personal use.

C) Personal comfort items, including smoking materials, notions and novelties, and confections.

D) Cosmetic and grooming items and services in excess of those for which payment is made under Medicaid or Medicare.

E) Personal clothing.

F) Personal reading matter.

G) Gifts purchased on behalf of a resident.

H) Flowers and plants.

I) Social events and entertainment offered outside the scope of the activities program, provided under Sec. 483.15(f) of this subpart.

J) Noncovered special care services such as privately hired nurses or aides.

K) Private room, except when therapeutically required (for example, isolation for infection control).

        L)   Specially prepared or alternative food requested instead of the food generally prepared by the facility, as required by Sec. 483.35 of this subpart.

    iii)   Requests for items and services.

        A)   The facility must not charge a resident (or his or her representative) for any item or service not requested by the resident.

        B)   The facility must not require a resident (or his or her representative) to request any item or service as a condition of admission or continued stay.

        C)   The facility must inform the resident (or his or her representative) requesting an item or service for which a charge will be made that there will be a charge for the item or service and what the charge will be.

d)   Free choice. The resident has the right to—

    1)   Choose a personal attending physician;

    2)   Be fully informed in advance about care and treatment and of any changes in that care or treatment that may affect the resident's well-being; and

    3)   Unless adjudged incompetent or otherwise found to be incapacitated under the laws of the State, participate in planning care and treatment or changes in care and treatment.

e)   Privacy and confidentiality. The resident has the right to personal privacy and confidentiality of his or her personal and clinical records.

    1)   Personal privacy includes accommodations, medical treatment, written and telephone communications, personal care, visits, and meetings of family and resident groups, but this does not require the facility to provide a private room for each resident;

    2)   Except as provided in paragraph (e)(3) of this section, the resident may approve or refuse the release of personal and clinical records to any individual outside the facility;

    3)   The resident's right to refuse release of personal and clinical records does not apply when—

        i)   The resident is transferred to another health care institution; or

        ii)   Record release is required by law.

f)   Grievances. A resident has the right to—

    1)   Voice grievances without discrimination or reprisal. Such grievances include those with respect to treatment which has been furnished as well as that which has not been furnished; and

    2)   Prompt efforts by the facility to resolve grievances the resident may have, including those with respect to the behavior of other residents.

g)   Examination of survey results. A resident has the right to—

    1)   Examine the results of the most recent survey of the facility conducted by Federal or State surveyors and any plan of correction in effect with respect to the facility. The facility must make the results available for examination in a place readily accessible to residents, and must post a notice of their availability; and

2) Receive information from agencies acting as client advocates, and be afforded the opportunity to contact these agencies.

h) Work. The resident has the right to—
1) Refuse to perform services for the facility;
2) Perform services for the facility, if he or she chooses, when—
   i) The facility has documented the need or desire for work in the plan of care;
   ii) The plan specifies the nature of the services performed and whether the services are voluntary or paid;
   iii) Compensation for paid services is at or above prevailing rates; and
   iv) The resident agrees to the work arrangement described in the plan of care.

i) Mail. The resident has the right to privacy in written communications, including the right to—
1) Send and promptly receive mail that is unopened; and
2) Have access to stationery, postage, and writing implements at the resident's own expense.

j) Access and visitation rights.
1) The resident has the right and the facility must provide immediate access to any resident by the following:
   i) Any representative of the Secretary;
   ii) Any representative of the State:
   iii) The resident's individual physician;
   iv) The State long term care ombudsman (established under section 307(a)(12) of the Older Americans Act of 1965);
   v) The agency responsible for the protection and advocacy system for developmentally disabled individuals (established under part C of the Developmental Disabilities Assistance and Bill of Rights Act);
   vi) The agency responsible for the protection and advocacy system for mentally ill individuals (established under the Protection and Advocacy for Mentally Ill Individuals Act);
   vii) Subject to the resident's right to deny or withdraw consent at any time, immediate family or other relatives of the resident; and
   viii) Subject to reasonable restrictions and the resident's right to deny or withdraw consent at any time, others who are visiting with the consent of the resident.
2) The facility must provide reasonable access to any resident by any entity or individual that provides health, social, legal, or other services to the resident, subject to the resident's right to deny or withdraw consent at any time.
3) The facility must allow representatives of the State Ombudsman, described in paragraph (j)(1)(iv) of this section, to examine a resident's clinical records with the permission of the resident or the resident's legal representative, and consistent with State law.

k) Telephone. The resident has the right to have reasonable access to the use of a telephone where calls can be made without being overheard.

l) Personal property. The resident has the right to retain and use personal possessions, including some furnishings, and appropriate clothing, as space permits, unless to do so would infringe upon the rights or health and safety of other residents.

m) Married couples. The resident has the right to share a room with his or her spouse when married residents live in the same facility and both spouses consent to the arrangement.

n) Self-Administration of Drugs. An individual resident may self-administer drugs if the interdisciplinary team, as defined by Sec. 483.20(d)(2)(ii), has determined that this practice is safe.

o) Refusal of certain transfers.

   1) An individual has the right to refuse a transfer to another room within the institution, if the purpose of the transfer is to relocate—
      i) A resident of a SNF from the distinct part of the institution that is a SNF to a part of the institution that is not a SNF, or
      ii) A resident of a NF from the distinct part of the institution that is a NF to a distinct part of the institution that is a SNF.
   2) A resident's exercise of the right to refuse transfer under paragraph (o) (1) of this section does not affect the individual's eligibility or entitlement to Medicare or Medicaid benefits.

Sec. 483.12 Admission, Transfer and Discharge Rights.

a) Transfer and discharge—

   1) Definition: Transfer and discharge includes movement of a resident to a bed outside of the certified facility whether that bed is in the same physical plant or not. Transfer and discharge does not refer to movement of a resident to a bed within the same certified facility.

   2) Transfer and discharge requirements. The facility must permit each resident to remain in the facility, and not transfer or discharge the resident from the facility unless—
      i) The transfer or discharge is necessary for the resident's welfare and the resident's needs cannot be met in the facility;
      ii) The transfer or discharge is appropriate because the resident's health has improved sufficiently so the resident no longer needs the services provided by the facility;
      iii) The safety of individuals in the facility is endangered;
      iv) The health of individuals in the facility would otherwise be endangered;
      v) The resident has failed, after reasonable and appropriate notice, to pay for (or to have paid under Medicare or Medicaid) a stay at the facility. For a resident who becomes eligible for Medicaid after admission to a facility, the facility may charge a resident only allowable charges under Medicaid; or
      vi) The facility ceases to operate.

3) Documentation. When the facility transfers or discharges a resident under any of the circumstances specified in paragraphs (a)(2)(i) through (v) of this section, the resident's clinical record must be documented. The documentation must be made by—

    i) The resident's physician when transfer or discharge is necessary under paragraph (a)(2)(i) or paragraph (a)(2)(ii) of this section; and

    ii) A physician when transfer or discharge is necessary under paragraph (a)(2)(iv) of this section.

4) Notice before transfer. Before a facility transfers or discharges a resident, the facility must—

    i) Notify the resident and, if known, a family member or legal representative of the resident of the transfer or discharge and the reasons for the move in writing and in a language and manner they understand.

    ii) Record the reasons in the resident's clinical record; and

    iii) Include in the notice the items described in paragraph (a)(6) of this section.

5) Timing of the notice.

    i) Except when specified in paragraph (a)(5)(ii) of this section, the notice of transfer or discharge required under paragraph (a)(4) of this section must be made by the facility at least 30 days before the resident is transferred or discharged.

    ii) Notice may be made as soon as practicable before transfer or discharge when—

        A) the safety of individuals in the facility would be endangered under paragraph (a)(2)(iii) of this section;

        B) The health of individuals in the facility would be endangered, under paragraph (a)(2)(iv) of this section;

        C) The resident's health improves sufficiently to allow a more immediate transfer or discharge, under paragraph (a)(2)(ii) of this section;

        D) An immediate transfer or discharge is required by the resident's urgent medical needs, under paragraph (a)(2)(i) of this section; or

        E) A resident has not resided in the facility for 30 days.

6) Contents of the notice. The written notice specified in paragraph (a)(4) of this section must include the following:

    i) The reason for transfer or discharge;

    ii) The effective date of transfer or discharge;

    iii) The location to which the resident is transferred or discharged;

    iv) A statement that the resident has the right to appeal the action to the State;

    v) The name, address and telephone number of the State long term care ombudsman;

    vi) For nursing facility residents with developmental disabilities, the mailing address and telephone number of the agency responsible for the protection and advocacy of developmentally disabled individuals established under Part C of the Developmental Disabilities Assistance and Bill of Rights Act; and

vii) For nursing facility residents who are mentally ill, the mailing address and telephone number of the agency responsible for the protection and advocacy of mentally ill individuals established under the Protection and Advocacy for Mentally Ill Individuals Act.

7) Orientation for transfer or discharge. A facility must provide sufficient preparation and orientation to residents to ensure safe and orderly transfer or discharge from the facility.

b) (b) Notice of bed-hold policy and readmission—

1) Notice before transfer. Before a nursing facility transfers a resident to a hospital or allows a resident to go on therapeutic leave, the nursing facility must provide written information to the resident and a family member or legal representative that specifies—

i) The duration of the bed-hold policy under the State plan, if any, during which the resident is permitted to return and resume residence in the nursing facility; and

ii) The nursing facility's policies regarding bed-hold periods, which must be consistent with paragraph (b)(3) of this section, permitting a resident to return.

2) Bed-hold notice upon transfer. At the time of transfer of a resident for hospitalization or therapeutic leave, a nursing facility must provide to the resident and a family member or legal representative written notice which specifies the duration of the bed-hold policy described in paragraph (b)(1) of this section.

3) Permitting resident to return to facility. A nursing facility must establish and follow a written policy under which a resident, whose hospitalization or therapeutic leave exceeds the bed-hold period under the State plan, is readmitted to the facility immediately upon the first availability of a bed in a semi-private room if the resident—

i) Requires the services provided by the facility; and

ii) Is eligible for Medicaid nursing facility services.

c) Equal access to quality care.

1) A facility must establish and maintain identical policies and practices regarding transfer, discharge, and the provision of services under the State plan for all individuals regardless of source of payment;

2) The facility may charge any amount for services furnished to non-Medicaid residents consistent with the notice requirement in Sec. 483.10(b)(5)(i) and (b)(6) describing the charges; and

3) The State is not required to offer additional services on behalf of a resident other than services provided in the State plan.

d) Admissions policy.

1) The facility must—

i) Not require residents or potential residents to waive their rights to Medicare or Medicaid; and

    ii)   Not require oral or written assurance that residents or potential residents are not eligible for, or will not apply for, Medicare or Medicaid benefits.

2)   The facility must not require a third party guarantee of payment to the facility as a condition of admission or expedited admission, or continued stay in the facility. However, the facility may require an individual who has legal access to a resident's income or resources available to pay for facility care to sign a contract, without incurring personal financial liability, to provide facility payment from the resident's income or resources.

3)   In the case of a person eligible for Medicaid, a nursing facility must not charge, solicit, accept, or receive, in addition to any amount otherwise required to be paid under the State plan, any gift, money, donation, or other consideration as a precondition of admission, expedited admission or continued stay in the facility. However,—

    i)   A nursing facility may charge a resident who is eligible for Medicaid for items and services the resident has requested and received, and that are not specified in the State plan as included in the term "nursing facility services" so long as the facility gives proper notice of the availability and cost of these services to residents and does not condition the resident's admission or continued stay on the request for and receipt of such additional services; and

    ii)   A nursing facility may solicit, accept, or receive a charitable, religious, or philanthropic contribution from an organization or from a person unrelated to a Medicaid eligible resident or potential resident, but only to the extent that the contribution is not a condition of admission, expedited admission, or continued stay in the facility for a Medicaid eligible resident.

4)   (4) States or political subdivisions may apply stricter admissions standards under State or local laws than are specified in this section, to prohibit discrimination against individuals entitled to Medicaid.

Sec. 483.13 Resident Behavior and Facility Practices.

a)   Restraints. The resident has the right to be free from any physical or chemical restraints imposed for purposes of discipline or convenience, and not required to treat the resident's medical symptoms.

b)   Abuse. The resident has the right to be free from verbal, sexual, physical, and mental abuse, corporal punishment, and involuntary seclusion.

c)   Staff treatment of residents. The facility must develop and implement written policies and procedures that prohibit mistreatment, neglect, and abuse of residents and misappropriation of resident property.

    1)   The facility must—

       i)   Not use verbal, mental, sexual, or physical abuse, corporal punishment, or involuntary seclusion;

       ii)   Not employ individuals who have been—

A)   Found guilty of abusing, neglecting, or mistreating residents by a court of law; or

B)   Have had a finding entered into the State nurse aide registry concerning abuse, neglect, mistreatment of residents or misappropriation of their property; and

iii) Report any knowledge it has of actions by a court of law against an employee, which would indicate unfitness for service as a nurse aide or other facility staff to the State nurse aide registry or licensing authorities.

2)   The facility must ensure that all alleged violations involving mistreatment, neglect, or abuse, including injuries of unknown source, and misappropriation of resident property are reported immediately to the administrator of the facility and to other officials in accordance with State law through established procedures (including to the State survey and certification agency).

3)   The facility must have evidence that all alleged violations are thoroughly investigated, and must prevent further potential abuse while the investigation is in progress.

4)   The results of all investigations must be reported to the administrator or his designated representative and to other officials in accordance with State law (including to the State survey and certification agency) within 5 working days of the incident, and if the alleged violation is verified appropriate corrective action must be taken.

Sec. 483.15 Quality of Life.

A facility must care for its residents in a manner and in an environment that promotes maintenance or enhancement of each resident's quality of life.

a)   Dignity. The facility must promote care for residents in a manner and in an environment that maintains or enhances each resident's dignity and respect in full recognition of his or her individuality.

b)   Self-determination and participation. The resident has the right to—

1)   Choose activities, schedules, and health care consistent with his or her interests, assessments, and plans of care;

2)   Interact with members of the community both inside and outside the facility; and

3)   Make choices about aspects of his or her life in the facility that are significant to the resident.

c)   Participation in resident and family groups.

1)   A resident has the right to organize and participate in resident groups in the facility;

2)   A resident's family has the right to meet in the facility with the families of other residents in the facility;

3)   The facility must provide a resident or family group, if one exists, with private space;

4)   Staff or visitors may attend meetings at the group's invitation;

5) The facility must provide a designated staff person responsible for providing assistance and responding to written requests that result from group meetings;

6) When a resident or family group exists, the facility must listen to the views and act upon the grievances and recommendations of residents and families concerning proposed policy and operational decisions affecting resident care and life in the facility.

d) Participation in other activities. A resident has the right to participate in social, religious, and community activities that do not interfere with the rights of other residents in the facility.

e) Accommodation of needs. A resident has the right to—

1) Reside and receive services in the facility with reasonable accommodation of individual needs and preferences, except when the health or safety of the individual or other residents would be endangered; and

2) Receive notice before the resident's room or roommate in the facility is changed.

f) Activities.

1) The facility must provide for an ongoing program of activities designed to meet, in accordance with the comprehensive assessment, the interests and the physical, mental, and psychosocial well-being of each resident.

2) The activities program must be directed by a qualified professional who—

   i) Is a qualified therapeutic recreation specialist or an activities professional who—

      A) Is licensed or registered, if applicable, by the State in which practicing; and

      B) Is eligible for certification as a therapeutic recreation specialist or as an activities professional by a recognized accrediting body on or after October 1, 1990; or

   ii) Has 2 years of experience in a social or recreational program within the last 5 years, 1 of which was full-time in a patient activities program in a health care setting; or

   iii) Is a qualified occupational therapist or occupational therapy assistant; or

   iv) Has completed a training course approved by the State.

g) Social Services.

1) The facility must provide medically-related social services to attain or maintain the highest practicable physical, mental, and psychosocial well-being of each resident.

2) A facility with more than 120 beds must employ a qualified social worker on a full-time basis.

3) Qualifications of social worker. A qualified social worker is an individual with—

   i) A bachelor's degree in social work or a bachelor's degree in a human services field including but not limited to sociology, special education, rehabilitation counseling, and psychology; and

        ii)   One year of supervised social work experience in a health care setting working directly with individuals.

h)   Environment. The facility must provide—

    1)   A safe, clean, comfortable, and homelike environment, allowing the resident to use his or her personal belongings to the extent possible;

    2)   Housekeeping and maintenance services necessary to maintain a sanitary, orderly, and comfortable interior;

    3)   Clean bed and bath linens that are in good condition;

    4)   Private closet space in each resident room, as specified in Sec. 483.70 (d)(2)(iv) of this part;

    5)   Adequate and comfortable lighting levels in all areas;

    6)   Comfortable and safe temperature levels. Facilities initially certified after October 1, 1990 must maintain a temperature range of 71-81 [deg]F; and

    7)   For the maintenance of comfortable sound levels.

SEC. 483.25 QUALITY OF CARE.

Each resident must receive and the facility must provide the necessary care and services to attain or maintain the highest practicable physical, mental, and psychosocial well-being, in accordance with the comprehensive assessment and plan of care.

a)   Activities of daily living. Based on the comprehensive assessment of a resident, the facility must ensure that—

    1)   A resident's abilities in activities of daily living do not diminish unless circumstances of the individual's clinical condition demonstrate that diminution was unavoidable. This includes the resident's ability to—

        i)   Bathe, dress, and groom;

        ii)   Transfer and ambulate;

        iii)   Toilet;

        iv)   Eat; and

        v)   Use speech, language, or other functional communication systems.

    2)   A resident is given the appropriate treatment and services to maintain or improve his or her abilities specified in paragraph (a)(1) of this section; and

    3)   A resident who is unable to carry out activities of daily living receives the necessary services to maintain good nutrition, grooming, and personal and oral hygiene.

b)   Vision and hearing. To ensure that residents receive proper treatment and assistive devices to maintain vision and hearing abilities, the facility must, if necessary, assist the resident—

    1)   In making appointments, and

    2)   By arranging for transportation to and from the office of a practitioner specializing in the treatment of vision or hearing impairment or the

office of a professional specializing in the provision of vision or hearing assistive devices.

c) Pressure sores. Based on the comprehensive assessment of a resident, the facility must ensure that—

   1) A resident who enters the facility without pressure sores does not develop pressure sores unless the individual's clinical condition demonstrates that they were unavoidable; and

   2) A resident having pressure sores receives necessary treatment and services to promote healing, prevent infection and prevent new sores from developing.

d) Urinary Incontinence. Based on the resident's comprehensive assessment, the facility must ensure that—

   1) A resident who enters the facility without an indwelling catheter is not catheterized unless the resident's clinical condition demonstrates that catheterization was necessary; and

   2) A resident who is incontinent of bladder receives appropriate treatment and services to prevent urinary tract infections and to restore as much normal bladder function as possible.

e) Range of motion. Based on the comprehensive assessment of a resident, the facility must ensure that—

   1) A resident who enters the facility without a limited range of motion does not experience reduction in range of motion unless the resident's clinical condition demonstrates that a reduction in range of motion is unavoidable; and

   2) A resident with a limited range of motion receives appropriate treatment and services to increase range of motion and/or to prevent further decrease in range of motion.

f) Mental and Psychosocial functioning. Based on the comprehensive assessment of a resident, the facility must ensure that—

   1) A resident who displays mental or psychosocial adjustment difficulty, receives appropriate treatment and services to correct the assessed problem, and

   2) A resident whose assessment did not reveal a mental or psychosocial adjustment difficulty does not display a pattern of decreased social interaction and/or increased withdrawn, angry, or depressive behaviors, unless the resident's clinical condition demonstrates that such a pattern was unavoidable.

g) Naso-gastric tubes. Based on the comprehensive assessment of a resident, the facility must ensure that—

   1) A resident who has been able to eat enough alone or with assistance is not fed by naso-gastric tube unless the resident's clinical condition demonstrates that use of a naso-gastric tube was unavoidable; and

   2) A resident who is fed by a naso-gastric or gastrostomy tube receives the appropriate treatment and services to prevent aspiration pneumonia, diarrhea, vomiting, dehydration, metabolic abnormalities, and nasal-pharyngeal ulcers and to restore, if possible, normal eating skills.

h) Accidents. The facility must ensure that—
    1) The resident environment remains as free of accident hazards as is possible; and(2) Each resident receives adequate supervision and assistance devices to prevent accidents.
i) Nutrition. Based on a resident's comprehensive assessment, the facility must ensure that a resident—
    1) Maintains acceptable parameters of nutritional status, such as body weight and protein levels, unless the resident's clinical condition demonstrates that this is not possible; and
    2) Receives a therapeutic diet when there is a nutritional problem.
j) Hydration. The facility must provide each resident with sufficient fluid intake to maintain proper hydration and health.
k) Special needs. The facility must ensure that residents receive proper treatment and care for the following special services:
    1) Injections;
    2) Parenteral and enteral fluids;
    3) Colostomy, ureterostomy, or ileostomy care;
    4) Tracheostomy care;
    5) Tracheal suctioning;
    6) Respiratory care;
    7) Foot care; and
    8) Prostheses.
l) Unnecessary drugs—
    1) General. Each resident's drug regimen must be free from unnecessary drugs. An unnecessary drug is any drug when used:
        i)   In excessive dose (including duplicate drug therapy); or
        ii)   For excessive duration; or
        iii) Without adequate monitoring; or
        iv)   Without adequate indications for its use; or
        v)   In the presence of adverse consequences which indicate the dose should be reduced or discontinued; or
        vi)   Any combinations of the reasons above.
    2) Antipsychotic Drugs. Based on a comprehensive assessment of a resident, the facility must ensure that—
        i)   Residents who have not used antipsychotic drugs are not given these drugs unless antipsychotic drug therapy is necessary to treat a specific condition as diagnosed and documented in the clinical record; and
        ii)   Residents who use antipsychotic drugs receive gradual dose reductions, and behavioral interventions, unless clinically contraindicated, in an effort to discontinue these drugs.
m) Medication Errors. The facility must ensure that—
    1) It is free of medication error rates of five percent or greater; and
    2) Residents are free of any significant medication errors.

[Source: Code of Federal Regulations, Title 42, Vol.3, From the U.S. Government Printing Office via GPO Access.]

Works Cited

Introduction

1. Mace NL and Rabins PV. *The 36-Hour Day*. Baltimore: Johns Hopkins University Press, 2006.

Chapter One

1. Cassels C. "Early Detection of Cognitive Impairment, Dementia Significantly Reduces Healthcare Costs," *Medscape Medical News*, July 20, 2010.

2. Talan J. "Changing the Definition of Dementia Could Improve Prevention and New Therapies," *Neurology Today*, January 2, 2009, p. 25.

3. Ibid.

4. Ibid.

5. Hamilton J. "Mad Cow and Alzheimer's Have Surprising Link," *NPR*, February 25, 2009. http://www.npr.org/templates/story/story.php?storyId=101145687 (accessed March 3, 2012).

6. Morley JE. "Alzheimer's Disease: Future Treatments," *Journal of the American Medical Directors Association*, 2011, 12(1): 1–7.

7. Saint Louis University, "Low Testosterone Linked to Alzheimer's Disease," *ScienceDaily*, October 5, 2010. http://www.sciencedaily.com/releases/2010/10/101005171202.htm (accessed March 3, 2012).

8. DeMarco B, "Nerve Growth Factor Study for Alzheimer's Disease (NGF)—CERE-110," *Alzheimer's Reading Room*, April 3, 2010. http://www.alzheimersreadingroom.com/2010/04/nerve-growth-factor-study-for.html (accessed March 3, 2012).

9. Swerdlow RH, Burns JM, and Khan SM. "The Alzheimer's Disease Mitochondrial Cascade Hypothesis," *J Alzheimers Dis*. 2010, 20(suppl 2): 265–279.

10. Fotuhi M. "How Accurate is Alzheimer's Diagnosis among Patients Over 80?" *Practical Neurology*, 2009, 8(8): 42–45.

11. Morley, "Alzheimer's Disease."

12. Lyketsos CG et al. "Mental and Behavioral Disturbances in Dementia: Findings from the Cache County Study on Memory in Aging," *American Journal of Psychiatry*, 2000, 157: 708–714.

13. Bermuda Hospitals Board, "Denial, Stigma Delaying Alzheimer's Diagnosis," *HealthDay News*, March 21, 2006. http://www.bermudahospitals.bm/health-wellness/MedicalNews.asp?chunkiid=113456 (accessed March 3, 2012).

14. Jacques G and Jacques A. *Understanding Dementia*. London: Harcourt Publishers, 2000.

15. Ibid.

16. State Government of Victoria, "Dementia: Coping with Placement," *BetterHealth Channel*, February 2011. http://www.betterhealth.vic.gov.au/bhcv2/bhcarticles.nsf/pages/Dementia_coping_with_placement (accessed March 3, 2012).

17. Ghent-Fuller J. "Understanding the Dementia Experience," *Alzheimer Society Cambridge*, September 27, 2003. http://www.alzheimer.guelph.org/downloads/12%20pt%20Understanding%20the%20Dementia%20Experience.pdf (accessed March 3, 2012).

18. National Highway Traffic and Safety Administration, "Current Screening and Assessment Practices," Community Mobility and Dementia DOT HS 810 864. http://www.nhtsa.dot.gov/people/injury/olddrive/commMobilityDementia/pages/CurrentScreening.htm (accessed March 3, 2012).

19. Foley JM. "The Experience of Being Demented," In RH Binstrock, SG Post, and PJ Whitehouse (Eds.), *Dementia and Aging: Ethics, Values and Policy Choices*. Baltimore: Johns Hopkins University Press, 1992: 30–43.

20. Latha KS. "The Noncompliant Patient in Psychiatry: The Case for and against Covert/Surreptitious Medication," *Psychopharmacology Today*, 2010, 8(1): 96–121.

21. Treloar A, Beats B, and Philpot M. "A Pill in the Sandwich: Covert Medication in Food and Drink," *Journal of the Royal Society of Medicine*. 2000, 93: 408–411.

22. McCurry S. *When a Family Member Has Dementia*. Westport, CT: Praeger Publishers, 2006.

23. Harris PB and Keady J. "Wisdom, Resilience and Successful Aging: Changing Public Discourses," *Dementia*, 2008, 7(1): 5–8.

24. Hilbert E. "Jim Valvano's ESPY Speech: Video, Transcript," *AOL News*, December 1, 2010. http://www.aolnews.com/2010/12/01/jim-valvanos-espys-speech-video-transcript/ (accessed March 3, 2012).

25. Jick H, Zornberg G, et al. "Statins and the Risk of Dementia," *Lancet*. 2000, 356 (9242): 1627–1631.

26. Zamrini E, McGwin G, and Roseman J. "Association between Statin Use and Alzheimer's Disease," *Neuroepidemiology*, 2004, 23: 94–98.

27. McGuinness B, Craig D, et al. Statins for the Prevention of Dementia," *Cochrane Database of Systematic Reviews*, 2009, Issue 2.

28. Ghent-Fuller. "Understanding."

29. Rockwood K et al. "Good Days and Bad Days in Dementia: A Qualitative Analysis of Variability in Symptom Expression," *Alzheimer's and Dementia*, 2009, 5(4): 233–234.

30. Cassels. "Early Detection."

31. Worcester S. "Lifestyle Changes Could Cut Alzheimer's Risk, Prevalence," *Internal Medicine News*, July 19, 2011. http://www.internalmedicinenews.com/news/print-friendly/lifestyle-changes-could-cut-alzheimer-s-risk-prevalence/d9a0376815.html?tx_ttnews%5BsViewPointer%5D=1 (accessed March 3, 2012).

CHAPTER TWO

1. Agronin ME. *How We Age.* Cambridge, MA: Da Capo Press, 2011.
2. "Unthinkable: The Alzheimer's Epidemic," Larry King Special, CNN, aired May 1, 2011.
3. Ibid.
4. Ibid.

CHAPTER THREE

1. *2011 Alzheimer's Disease Facts and Figures,* http://www.alz.org/downloads/Facts_Figures_2011.pdf (accessed September 28, 2011).
2. Norton M, Smith K, et al. "Greater Risk of Dementia when Spouse Has Dementia? The Cache County Study," *Journal of the American Geriatrics Society,* 2010, 58(5): 895–900.
3. Wang S. "How Depression Weakens the Brain," *Wall Street Journal,* July 3, 2007, http://online.wsj.com/article/SB118342335959256070-search.html.
4. http://www.memorylossdvd.com/ (accessed September 28, 2011).
5. Schulz R, Burgio L, et al. "Resources for Enhancing Alzheimer's Caregiver Health (REACH): Overview, Site-Specific Outcomes, and Future Directions," *Gerontologist,* 2003, 43(4): 514–520.
6. Meyer H. "Housing Bust Derails Some Seniors' Assisted Living Care," *Kaiser Health News,* August 21, 2011.http://www.kaiserhealthnews.org/Stories/2011/August/22/housing-crash-assisted-living.aspx (accessed March 3, 2012).
7. http://www.time.com/time/politics/article/0,8599,1946431,00.html (accessed September 29, 2011).
8. http://www.kintera.org/atf/cf/%7BB96E2E84-AF7D-4656-9C86-285306F00E19%7D/2011%20HOPE%20for%20Alz%20Fact%20Sheet.pdf (accessed September 29, 2011).

CHAPTER FOUR

1. The History of Nursing Home, http://www.4fate.org/history.html (accessed May 2, 2012).
2. Nursing Homes: History, http://medicine.jrank.org/pages/1243/Nursing-Homes-History.html (accessed September 22, 2011).
3. Feng Z, Fennell M, et al. "Growth of Racial and Ethnic Minorities in US Nursing Homes Driven by Demographics and Possible Disparities in Options," *Health Affairs,* 2011, 30(7): 1358–1365.
4. Alzheimer's Disease Facts and Figures, http://www.alz.org/downloads/Facts_Figures_2011.pdf (accessed September 22, 2011).
5. The Senior Care Source: Facts, Figures, and Forecasts, "Skilled Nursing Facilities in a Changing World," *Novartis,* 2008, 5: 21.
6. Alzheimer A. "Uber eine eigenartige erkrankung der hirnrinde," Allgemeine Zeitschrift fur Psychiatrie und Psychisch-Gerichtliche Medizin, 1907, 64: 146–148.
7. Hall RCW, Hall RCW, and Chapman M. "Nursing Home Violence: Occurrence, Risks, and Interventions," *Annals of Long-Term Care,* 2009, 17(1): 25–39.

8. Fitzwater EL and Gates DM. "Testing an Intervention to Reduce Assaults on Nursing Assistants in Nursing Homes: A Pilot Study," *Geriatric Nursing*, 2002, 23: 18–23.

9. Castle NG and Engberg J. "Organizational Characteristics Associated with Staff Turnover in Nursing Homes," *Gerontologist*, 2006, 46(1): 62–73.

10. Tucker ME. "Resident-Resident Conflicts Are Subjects of Study, Concern," *Caring for the Ages*, 2009, 10(5): 1.

11. http://www.caremedia.cs.cmu.edu (accessed September 23, 2011).

12. Pearce BW. *Senior Living Communities: Operations Management and Marketing for Assisted Living, Congregate, and Continuing Care Retirement Communities*. Baltimore: Johns Hopkins University Press, 1998.

13. Tucker ME. "Resident-Resident Conflicts," 14.

14. Bern-Klug M et al. "Characteristics of Nursing Home Social Services Directors: How Common Is a Degree in Social Work?" *Journal of the American Medical Directors Association*, 2009, 10(1): 36–44.

15. Parker-Oliver D and Kurzejeski LS. "Nursing Home Social Services: Policy and Practice," *Journal of Gerontologic Social Work*, 2004, 42: 37–50.

16. Bern-Klug M et al. "Characteristics of Nursing Home Social Services Directors."

17. Schor JD. *The Nursing Home Guide*. New York: Berkley, 2008, p. 139.

18. Ballard C and Waite J. "The Effectiveness of Atypical Antipsychotics for the Treatment of Aggression and Psychosis in Alzheimer's Disease," *Cochrane Database Syst Rev*, 2006, (1): CD003476.

19. http://www.guideline.gov/content.aspx?id=11533 (accessed March 3, 2012).

20. Westerberg RK. "Choosing a Nursing Home," *AARP Magazine*, 2007. http://bishopdaviescenter.com/?page_id=87 (accessed March 3, 2012).

21. http://www.longtermcareliving.com/pdf/myths.pdf (accessed September 23, 2011).

22. Chillala J and Sinclair A. "Quality of Medical Care in British Care Homes," *Journal of the American Medical Association*, 2009, 10(4): 224.

CHAPTER FIVE

1. The Senior Care Source: Facts, Figures, and Forecasts. "Assisted Living: Diverse Sector Evolves," *Novartis*, 2008, 5: 40.

2. Cartwright JC, Miller L, and Volpin M. "Hospice in Assisted Living: Promoting Good Quality Care at End of Life," *Gerontologist*, 2009, 49(4): 508–516.

3. The Senior Care Source. "Assisted Living."

4. Hawes C and Phillips C. "Defining Quality in Assisted Living: Comparing Apples, Oranges, and Broccoli," *Gerontologist*, 2007, 47(suppl 1): 40–50.

5. The Senior Care Source. "Assisted Living."

6. Solari S, Brown B, and Eaton J, "Conflicts, Friendship Cliques and Territorial Displays in Senior Center Environments," *Journal of Aging Studies*, 2006, 20(3): 237–252.

7. http://www.azcentral.com/community/chandler/articles/2010/12/28/20101228chandler-woman-bullied-at-retirement-community.html (accessed September 24, 2011).

8. http://money.cnn.com/galleries/2009/moneymag/0902/gallery.continuing_care.moneymag/index.html (accessed September 24, 2011).

9. The Senior Care Source. "Assisted Living."

10. Magsi H and Malloy T. "Underrecognition of Cognitive Impairment in Assisted Living Facilities," *J Am Geriatr Soc*, 2005, 53(2): 295–298.

11. Alzheimer's Disease Facts and Figures, http://www.alz.org/downloads/Facts_Figures_2011.pdf (accessed September 24, 2011).

12. Rosenblatt A, Samus QM, et al. "The Maryland Assisted Living Study: Prevalence, Recognition and Treatment of Dementia and Other Psychiatric Disorders in the Assisted Living Population of Central Maryland," *J Am Geriatr Soc*, 2004, 52: 1618–1625.

13. Hawes C, Phillips C, et al. "A National Survey of Assisted Living Facilities," *Gerontologist*, 2003, 43(6): 875–882.

14. http://www.alz.org/national/documents/prevalence_Alz_assist.pdf (accessed September 25, 2011).

15. Wagenaar D, Mickus M, et al. "An Administrator's Perspective on Mental Health in Assisted Living," *Psychiatric Services*, 2003, 54(December): 1644–1646.

16. http://www.ahcancal.org/ncal/resources/Documents/2011AssistedLivingRegulatoryReview.pdf (accessed September 25, 2011).

CHAPTER SIX

1. http://www.nadsa.org/ (accessed September 29, 2011).

2. The Senior Care Source: Facts, Figures, and Forecasts. "Home Healthcare and Family Caregiving," *Novartis*, 2008, 5: 45.

3. http://www.caremanager.org/ (accessed September 29, 2011).

4. http://www.nytimes.com/2010/05/05/us/05search.html (accessed September 28, 2011).

5. http://www.alz.org/comfortzone/ (accessed September 29, 2011).

6. http://www.emfinders.com/ (accessed September 29, 2011).

7. http://www.lojacksafetynet.com/bringthemback/ (accessed September 30, 2011).

8. http://www.alz.org/safetycenter/we_can_help_safety_medicalert_safereturn.asp (accessed September 29, 2011).

CHAPTER SEVEN

1. Used by permission of McLean Hospital. http://www.mclean.harvard.edu/patient/geriatrics/gnu.php (accessed September 25, 2011).

2. http://www.msnbc.msn.com/id/44707138/ns/health-aging/#.ToS_uXMx_GA (accessed September 28, 2011).

3. http://abclocal.go.com/wabc/story?section=news/local8id=6755111 (accessed December 31, 2009).

4. Bang J, Price D, et al. "ECT Treatment for Two Cases of Dementia-Related Pathological Yelling," *J Neuropsychiatry Clin Neurosci*, 2008, 20(3): 379.

5. Groulx B. "Screaming and Wailing in Dementia Patients: Part 1," *Canadian Alzheimer Disease Review*, January 2004, 11–14.

6. Becker R and Lindesay J. "Institutional Care." In S Gauthier (Ed.), *Clinical Diagnosis and Management of Alzheimer's Disease* (2nd ed.). Boston: Butterworth-Heinemann, 1999, p. 336.

7. http://www.bhconcepts.com/asp/faq/faq.asp?m=6#5 (accessed September 25, 2011).

8. Yazgan I, Greenwald B, et al. "Geriatric Psychiatry versus General Psychiatry Inpatient Treatment of the Elderly," *Am J Psychiatry,* 2004, 161: 352–355.

CHAPTER EIGHT

1. Lindesay J. "Memory Clinics." In R Jacoby, C Oppenheimer, et al., eds. *Oxford Textbook of Old Age Psychiatry.* New York: Oxford University Press, 2008.
2. Ibid.
3. Lindesay. "Memory Clinics."
4. McNamara D. "Modified Mental-State Exam More Accurate," *Caring for the Ages,* November 2010, p. 20.
5. Lindesay. "Memory Clinics."
6. http://newsvote.bbc.co.uk/2/hi/health/7853697.stm (accessed September 25, 2011).
7. http://newsvote.bbc.co.uk/2/hi/health/7865494.stm (accessed September 25, 2011).
8. Coombes R. "Evidence Lacking for Memory Clinics to Tackle Dementia, Say Critics," *British Medical Journal,* 2009, 338:b550.
9. http://www.nytimes.com/2010/11/26/health/26alzheimers.html?_r=1 (accessed September 26, 2011).
10. Mattson N, et al. "CSF Biomarkers and Incipient Alzheimer Disease in Patients with Mild Cognitive Impairment," *JAMA,* 2009, 302(4): 385–393.
11. Petersen RC and Trojanowski JQ. "Use of Alzheimer Disease Biomarkers: Potentially Yes for Clinical Trials but Not Yet for Clinical Practice," *JAMA,* 2009, 302(4): 436.
12. http://www.alzheimersassociation.org/alzheimers_disease_clinical_studies.asp (accessed March 3, 2012).
13. http://www.nia.nih.gov/alzheimers/publication/participating-alzheimers-disease -clinical-trials-and-studies-fact-sheet (accessed March 3, 2012).
14. http://www.focr.org/new-york-times-lack-of-study-volunteers-hobbles-cancer -fight.html (accessed September 26, 2011).
15. Jolley D. "Memory Clinics and Dementia Care: The Issue is Stigma Not Screening," *British Medical Journal,* 2009, 338:b550.

CHAPTER NINE

1. http://www.whitehead-elderlaw.com/sitebuildercontent/sitebuilderfiles/ texaslegalstandardsrelated-final-rev.pdf (accessed September 26, 2011).
2. Ganzini L, Volicer L, et al., "Ten Myths About Decision-Making Capacity," *J Am Med Dir Assoc,* 2004. 5: 263–267.
3. http://online.wsj.com/article/SB124520056162621509.html (accessed September 26, 2011).
4. http://www.medscape.com/viewarticle/709333 (accessed September 26, 2011).
5. http://www.probatelawyerblog.com/2009/10/brooke-astors-son-found-guilty. html (accessed September 26, 2011).
6. http://www.usatoday.com/news/nation/2006-07-28-astor_x.htm (accessed March 3, 2012).

7. http://www.nytimes.com/2009/08/18/nyregion/18astor.html (accessed September 26, 2011).

8. http://www.nypost.com/p/news/local/manhattan/item_Zxqt1cuZkD09owbhQK oIYO (accessed September 26, 2011).

9. http://209.240.158.192/wp-content/uploads/2010/06/02_March_April_2010.pdf (accessed September 26, 2011).

10. http://online.wsj.com/article/SB10001424052748704681904576315662838 806984.html (accessed September 26, 2011).

11. http://money.cnn.com/2011/08/10/retirement/protecting_parents.moneymag/ index.htm (accessed September 26, 2011).

CHAPTER TEN

1. http://books.nap.edu/openbook.php?record_id=12089 (accessed September 26, 2011).

2. http://www.msnbc.msn.com/id/5868712/ns/health-aging/t/ageism-america/ (accessed September 26, 2011).

CHAPTER ELEVEN

1. Ready R and Ott B. "Quality of Life Measures for Dementia," *Health and Quality of Life Outcomes*, 2003, 1: 11.

2. http://www.bellaonline.com/articles/art23319.asp (accessed September 26, 2011).

3. Norton M, Smith K, et al. "Spousal Dementia Caregiving as a Risk Factor for Incident Dementia?" *Alzheimer's & Dementia*, 2009, 5(4): 380–381.

4. http://online.wsj.com/article/SB10001424052748704471504574449572778 372770.html (accessed March 3, 2012).

5. http://www.ahcancal.org/News/publication/Provider/CoverNov2009.pdf (accessed September 26, 2011).

6. Devere R. "Highlights from the International Alzheimer's Disease Conference," *Practical Neurology,* October 2009: 49.

7. http://online.wsj.com/article/SB10001424052748704538404574540163096944766.html (accessed September 26, 2011).

APPENDIX

1. http://www.nytimes.com/2008/09/30/us/30nursing.html (accessed October 9, 2011).

Suggested Resources

About.com Alzheimer's Site: www.alzheimers.about.com
Administration on Aging: www.aoa.gov
Alzheimer Research Forum: www.alzforum.org
Alzheimer's Association: www.alz.org
Alzheimer's Association Online Community: http://alzheimers.infopop.cc/eve/ubb.x
Alzheimer's Association Trial Match: http://www.alz.org/research/clinical_trials/find
    _clinical_trials_trialmatch.asp
Alzheimer's Disease Education and Referral (ADEAR) Center: www.nia.nih.gov/
    alzheimers
Alzheimer's Disease International: www.alz.co.uk
Alzheimer's Disease.com: www.alzheimersdisease.com
Alzheimer's Foundation of America: www.alzfdn.org
Alzheimer's Prevention: www.alzprevention.org
Alzheimer's Society: www.alzheimers.org.uk
American Association for Geriatric Psychiatry: www.aagponline.org
Aricept Site: www.aricept.com
Assisted Living Federation of America: www.alfa.org
Children of Aging Parents: www.caps4caregivers.org
Ethnic Elders Care: www.ethnicelderscare.net
Exelon Patch Site: www.exelonpatch.com
Family Caregiver Alliance: www.caregiver.org
Financial Planning Association: www.fpanet.org
Fisher Center for Alzheimer's Research Foundation: www.alzinfo.org
Leading Age: www.aahsa.org
Mayo Clinic Alzheimer's Site: www.mayoclinic.com/health/alzheimers/AZ99999
Medicare: www.medicare.gov
Medicare Nursing Home Compare: www.medicare.gov/nhcompare
Mind in Memory Care: www.mindinmemorycare.com
Moving in Nurturing Directions (MIND) in Memory Care: http://www.mindinmemory
    care.com/
Namenda Site: www.namenda.com

National Academy of Elder Law Attorneys: www.naela.org
National Adult Day Services Association: www.nadsa.org
National Alliance for Caregiving: www.caregiving.org
National Association of Area Agencies on Aging: www.n4a.org
National Association of Professional Geriatric Care Managers: www.caremanager.org
National Consumer Voice for Long-Term Care: http://www.theconsumervoice.org/
National Council of Certified Dementia Practitioners: www.nccdp.org
National Elder law Foundation: www.nelf.org
National Family Caregiver's Association: www.thefamilycaregiver.org
National Long-Term Care Ombudsman Resource Center: http://www.ltcombudsman.org
National Memory Screening: www.nationalmemoryscreening.org
Razadyne ER Site: www.razadyneer.com
Senior Decision: www.seniordecision.com

INDEX

About the Author

ANDREW S. ROSENZWEIG, MD, MPH, is considered one of the foremost experts on treating dementia and on increasing the quality of life for patients and caregivers. He is a board-certified geriatric psychiatrist who has worked in the fields of dementia and long-term care since completing his fellowship training in Geriatric Psychiatry in 1996. He has a Masters of Public Health degree in Epidemiology and has worked in multiple settings relevant to this topic, including home-care, office-based care, general and psychiatric hospitals, assisted living facilities, and nursing homes. Presently he is Chief Clinical Officer for MedOptions, the largest provider of behavioral health services to nursing home and assisted living facility residents in Connecticut, Massachusetts, Rhode Island, Pennsylvania, Maryland and New Jersey. MedOptions serves over 25,000 residents in 400 facilities through a staff of 250 clinicians. As Chief Clinical Officer, he collaborates with advanced practice nurses, physician assistants, psychologists, and licensed clinical social workers. He is also an assistant clinical professor in the Department of Psychiatry and Human Behavior at Brown University. He received a 2007 Teaching Recognition Award from the Warren Alpert Medical School of Brown University. In 2010 he was the Alzheimer's site guide for About.com, a New York Times company. He has participated in and testified at numerous court hearings involving legal guardianship and mental capacity, and he has lectured frequently on issues involving late-life mental health and dementia. He has led support groups in nursing homes and assisted living facilities, and he has provided numerous inservice educational programs to facility staff. Most importantly, though, he's learned that while the best outcomes often involve trial and error, nothing predicts success more than listening, attempting to understand what others (patients, staff, and caregivers alike) are trying to communicate, and respecting their beliefs and opinions.

About the Series Editor

JULIE SILVER, MD, is Assistant Professor, Harvard Medical School, Department of Physical Medicine and Rehabilitation, and is on the medical staff at Brigham & Women's, Massachusetts General and Spaulding Rehabilitation Hospitals in Boston, Massachusetts. Dr. Silver has authored, edited or co-edited dozens of book, including medical textbooks and consumer health guides. She is also the Chief Editor of Books at Harvard Health Publications. Dr. Silver has won many awards including the American Medical Writers Association Solimene Award for Excellence in Medical Writing and the prestigious Lane Adams Quality of Life Award from the American Cancer Society. Silver is active teaching health care providers how to write and publish, and she is the Director of an annual course offered by the Harvard Medical School Department of Continuing Education titled "Publishing Books, Memoirs and Other Creative Non-Fiction." For more about her work, visit www.JulieSilverMD.com.